SBAs, EMQs & SAQs in
SURGERY

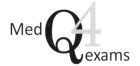

Med Q4 exams

Matthew Hanks

tfm Publishing Limited, Castle Hill Barns, Harley, Shrewsbury, SY5 6LX, UK
Tel: +44 (0)1952 510061; Fax: +44 (0)1952 510192
E-mail: info@tfmpublishing.com; Web site: www.tfmpublishing.com

Editing, design & typesetting: Nikki Bramhill BSc Hons Dip Law
Cover photo: © iStock.com
Medical team preparing equipment for surgery (ShutterOK) — Stock photo ID: 507756350

First edition: © 2019
Paperback   ISBN: 978-1-910079-75-1
E-book editions: © 2019
epub   ISBN: 978-1-910079-76-8
Mobi   ISBN: 978-1-910079-77-5
Web pdf   ISBN: 978-1-910079-78-2

Printed by Gutenberg Press Ltd., Gudja Road, Tarxien, GXQ 2902, Malta
Tel: +356 2398 2201; Fax: +356 2398 2290
E-mail: info@gutenberg.com.mt; Web site: www.gutenberg.com.mt

Contents

About the Editor

Dr. Matthew Hanks graduated from the University of Sheffield in 2015 with an MBChB in medicine; prior to this Matthew studied for a BSc Biomedical Science degree in Sheffield graduating in 2010 with a first class honours degree. He has a keen interest in teaching and has devised many different teaching programmes for students which have been engaging and received positive feedback. He now hopes to take this passion further by providing students with resources that are both useful and informative to enhance their learning opportunities.

Contributors

Miss Rose Gnap BSc (Hons) BMBS PGCert MRCSEd
CT2 Core Surgical Trainee, East Midlands North Deanery

Dr. Matthew Hanks BSc (Hons) MBChB PG Cert Surgery
CT2 Core Surgical Trainee, East Midlands North Deanery

Dr. Richard Harrold MBChB (Hons)
Locum Senior House Officer, South Yorkshire Region

Dr. Mei-Ling Henry BMedSci BMBS
CT2 Core Surgical Trainee, East Midlands North Deanery

Dr. Chloe Theodorou BMBS
CT1 Core Surgical Trainee, North Western Deanery

Dr. Emma Whitehall BMedSci MBChB (Hons)
CT2 Core Surgical Trainee, East Midlands North Deanery

Acknowledgements

I would like to thank all those who have taken the time to contribute to this title which is the amalgamation of knowledge from professionals studying and working all over the United Kingdom; without their hard work and dedication, this book would not have been possible.

I would like to thank Megan Ward and Glenda Hanks for their patience whilst the book has taken shape and the many nights of proof reading the text to ensure it will be useful for students. Koda and Joel Ward have provided a useful distraction when required!

Finally, the road to medical finals is a long one and this is the last major hurdle to becoming a doctor; the many hours of hard work and dedication already demonstrated in getting this far is about to pay off. All that is left to say is good luck!

Matthew Hanks
June 2019

Normal reference values

Please note normal reference values may vary between different hospitals.

Hb	Male 131-166g/L
	Female 110-147g/L
MCV	81-96fL
Platelets	150-400 x 10^9/L
WCC	3.5-9.5 x 10^9/L
Neutrophils	1.7-6.5 x 10^9/L
Lymphocytes	1.0-3.0 x 10^9/L
Eosinophils	0.04-0.5 x 10^9/L
Basophils	0.0-0.25 x 10^9/L
Sodium	133-146mmol/L
Potassium	3.5-5.3mmol/L
Urea	2.5-7.8mmol/L
Creatinine	62-106μmol/L
eGFR	>90
Calcium	2.25-2.5mmol/L
Total protein	60-80g/L
Globulin	18-36g/L
Bilirubin	0-21μmol/L
ALT	0-41iU/L
ALP	30-130iU/L

AST	0-35iU/L
Albumin	35-50g/L
PT	10.1-11.8 seconds
APTT	20.2-28.7 seconds
Thrombin time	11.3-17.4 seconds
Fibrinogen	2.0-4.0g/L
CRP	0-5mg/L

Abbreviations

AAA	Abdominal aortic aneurysm
ABG	Arterial blood gas
ABPI	Ankle Brachial Pressure Index
ACE	Angiotensin-converting enzyme
ACL	Anterior cruciate ligament
ACTH	Adrenocorticotrophic hormone
ADH	Antidiuretic hormone
AF	Atrial fibrillation
AFP	α-fetoprotein
AKI	Acute kidney injury
ALP	Alkaline phosphatase
ALT	Alanine aminotransferase
APACHE II	Acute Physiology and Chronic Health Evaluation II
APTT	Activated partial thromboplastin time
ARDS	Acute respiratory distress syndrome
AST	Aspartate aminotransferase
ATP	Adenosine triphosphate
BDI	Beck Depression Inventory
BP	Blood pressure
BPM	Beats per minute
CA19-9	Carbohydrate antigen 19-9
CBD	Common bile duct
Cl⁻	Chloride
CNS	Central nervous system
COPD	Chronic obstructive pulmonary disease
CPR	Cardiopulmonary resuscitation

CRP	C-reactive protein
CSF	Cerebrospinal fluid
CT	Computed tomography
CTPA	Computed tomography pulmonary angiography
CT KUB	Computed tomography of the kidney, ureters and bladder
CVA	Cerebrovascular accident
CXR	Chest X-ray
DHS	Dynamic hip screw
DIC	Disseminated intravascular coagulation
DKA	Diabetic ketoacidosis
DMARD	Disease-modifying anti-rheumatic drug
DNACPR	Do not attempt cardiopulmonary resuscitation
DVT	Deep vein thrombosis
EBV	Epstein-Barr virus
ECG	Electrocardiogram
EEG	Electroencephalogram
ENT	Ear, nose and throat
ERCP	Endoscopic retrograde cholangiopancreatography
ESR	Erythrocyte sedimentation rate
EVAR	Endovascular aneurysm repair
FAP	Familial adenomatous polyposis
FBC	Full blood count
FiO_2	Fraction of inspired oxygen
FSH	Follicle-stimulating hormone
GCS	Glasgow Coma Scale
GFR	Glomerular filtration rate
GH	Growth hormone
GI	Gastrointestinal
GORD	Gastro-oesophageal reflux disease
GTN	Glyceryl trinitrate
HADS	Hospital Anxiety and Depression Scale
Hb	Haemoglobin
HCl^-	Hydrogen chloride

HIV	Human immunodeficiency virus
HNPCC	Hereditary non-polyposis colon cancer
HPV	Human papilloma virus
HRT	Hormone replacement therapy
IBD	Inflammatory bowel disease
ICP	Intracranial pressure
Ig	Immunoglobulin
IIH	Idiopathic intracranial hypertension
IM	Intramuscular
INR	International Normalised Ratio
IV	Intravenous
IVC	Inferior vena cava
JVP	Jugular venous pressure
K^+	Potassium
KUB	Kidney, ureter, bladder
LDH	Lactate dehydrogenase
LFT	Liver function test
LH	Luteinising hormone
LUTS	Lower urinary tract symptoms
MAOI	Monoamine oxidase inhibitors
MCL	Medial collateral ligament
MCV	Mean corpuscular volume
MDT	Multidisciplinary team
MEN	Multiple endocrine neoplasia
MI	Myocardial infarction
MRCP	MR cholangiopancreatography
MRI	Magnetic resonance imaging
MSU	Midstream urine
Na^+	Sodium
NaOH	Sodium hydroxide
NG	Nasogastric
NICE	The National Institute for Health and Care Excellence
NSAID	Non-steroidal anti-inflammatory drug

OGD	Oesophagogastroduodenoscopy
OME	Otitis media with effusion
ORIF	Open reduction and internal fixation
OTC	On-table cholangiogram
PCL	Posterior cruciate ligament
PE	Pulmonary embolism
PET	Positron emission tomography
PHQ-9	Patient Health Questionnaire
POP	Plaster of Paris
PPI	Proton pump inhibitor
PSA	Prostate-specific antigen
PT	Prothrombin time
PTH	Parathyroid hormone
SAH	Subarachnoid haemorrhage
SCC	Squamous cell carcinoma
SDH	Subdural haemorrhage
SIADH	Syndrome of inappropriate antidiuretic hormone
SIRS	Systemic inflammatory response syndrome
SLE	Systemic lupus erythematosus
SSRI	Selective serotonin reuptake inhibitor
TB	Tuberculosis
TCA	Tricyclic antidepressant
TCC	Transitional cell carcinoma
TIA	Transient ischaemic attack
TNM	Tumour, nodes and metastasis
TSH	Thyroid-stimulating hormone
TURP	Transurethral resection of the prostate
U&Es	Urea & electrolytes
USS	Ultrasound scan
UTI	Urinary tract infection
VTE	Venous thromboembolism
WCC	White cell count

Section 1

Questions

Chapter 1

Upper GI surgery
QUESTIONS

Single best answer questions

1) A 42-year-old female with known gallstones presents to the emergency department with epigastric pain radiating to the back. The pain started 24 hours ago and is severe in nature. Bloods reveal an amylase at 2000IU/L. What is the most likely diagnosis?

a. Acute pancreatitis.
b. Ascending cholangitis.
c. Chronic pancreatitis.
d. Biliary colic.

2) An 82-year-old male is brought to the emergency department by paramedics following several episodes of haematemesis at home. He is hypotensive and tachycardic. He has a previous history of endovascular repair of an AAA. What condition must be excluded as a cause of this patient's haematemesis?

a. Aorto-enteric fistula.
b. Mallory-Weiss tear.
c. Gastro-oesophageal reflux disease.
d. Gastritis.

3) A 42-year-old female presents to the surgical assessment unit with a 24-hour history of right upper quadrant pain radiating to the right shoulder. On examination, she is tender in the right upper quadrant with a positive Murphy's sign. There is no evidence of jaundice. Bloods show a raised WCC and CRP. Liver function tests are unremarkable. What is the most likely diagnosis?

a. Ascending cholangitis.
b. Biliary colic.
c. Acute cholangitis.
d. Choledochal cyst.

4) A 67-year-old male presents to the emergency department with a 48-hour history of vomiting and abdominal pain. He has noted abdominal distention and in the last 24 hours has not opened his bowels or passed any flatus. On examination, he has a distended abdomen and auscultation reveals tinkling bowel sounds. An abdominal X-ray shows central, dilated loops of bowel with valvulae conniventes present on these loops. What is the most likely diagnosis?

a. Duodenal atresia.
b. Bacterial gastroenteritis.
c. Large bowel obstruction.
d. Small bowel obstruction.

5) A 45-year-old male presents to the emergency department with a 24-hour history of vomiting, abdominal pain and constipation. He has not passed any flatus during this time. He has a past medical history of gallstones, previous open repair of a duodenal ulcer and Type 1 diabetes mellitus. On examination, his abdomen is distended and bowel sounds are decreased. Abdominal X-ray shows evidence of a small bowel obstruction with pneumobilia. What is the most likely cause of this patient's small bowel obstruction?

a. Gastric volvulus.
b. Gallstone ileus.
c. Adhesions.
d. Gastrointestinal stromal tumour.

6) A 56-year-old male is admitted to the surgical assessment unit with a 36-hour history of right upper quadrant pain and vomiting. The pain is worse following food and he has been unable to eat anything for 24 hours. On examination, he has right upper quadrant tenderness but no other findings. Blood results show a raised WCC and CRP. The clerking doctor believes this patient may have acute cholecystitis. What is the most appropriate next investigation to request for this patient?

a. Ultrasound abdomen.
b. MRCP.
c. ERCP.
d. Abdominal X-ray.

7) A 56-year-old male presents to the outpatient clinic with a 4-week history of dysphagia. He has had a feeling of a lump in his throat for the past 3 weeks and has had several episodes of regurgitating food. On examination, a prominent lump is seen on swallowing and the patient appears to take a double swallow. A barium swallow confirms the diagnosis. What is the most likely diagnosis?

a. Oesophageal perforation.
b. Pharyngeal pouch.
c. Oesophageal web.
d. Achalasia.

8) A 42-year-old female presents to the surgical outpatient clinic with a 12-week history of dyspepsia which is worst when lying flat and has not settled with a trial of proton pump inhibitor therapy. She has experienced issues with regurgitating food soon after eating several times over the past 5 weeks which is distressing her. An oesophago-gastroduodenoscopy (OGD) is performed which shows an upward displacement of the gastro-oesophageal junction. What is the underlying diagnosis?

a. Barrett's oesophagus.
b. Gastro-oesophageal reflux disease.
c. Sliding hiatus hernia.
d. Rolling hiatus hernia.

9) A 67-year-old female presents to the outpatient surgical clinic with a 6-week history of vague abdominal pain, nausea and diarrhoea. She believes her clothes feel looser than previously and her friends have commented that she

has a flushed appearance. Blood results show a raised serotonin level. What is the underlying diagnosis?

a. Carcinoid.
b. Gastrointestinal stromal tumour.
c. Cholangiocarcinoma.
d. Gallbladder empyema.

10) A 45-year-old female presents to the emergency department with right upper quadrant pain, lethargy and fever. She had a recent hospital admission in which she was treated for acute cholecystitis. Observations in the department show a tachycardia and swinging pyrexia. Blood results show a raised WCC and CRP. LFTs were unremarkable. What is the underlying diagnosis?

a. Hepatitis A.
b. Gallbladder empyema.
c. Cholangiocarcinoma.
d. Liver abscess.

11) A 42-year-old male undergoes a laparotomy for removal of a gastrointestinal malignancy. The operation is successful and the histological report notes it is a mesenchymal neoplasm of the gastrointestinal tract arising from the interstitial cells of Cajal. Further analysis of the tumour shows a mutation in the c-KIT gene. What is the most likely diagnosis?

a. Carcinoid.
b. Gastrointestinal stromal tumour.
c. Cholangiocarcinoma.
d. Lipoma.

12) A 56-year-old female presents to her local emergency department with sudden-onset epigastric pain radiating to her back relieved when sitting forwards. She is known to have gallstones. Bloods and imaging confirm a diagnosis of pancreatitis. On examination, she has moderate bruising to her flanks. What is the name of this sign?

a. Psoas.
b. Cullen.
c. Grey-Turner.
d. Rovsing's.

13) A 25-year-old male is admitted to the emergency department with sudden-onset pain in his chest, neck and upper abdomen. He is hypotensive and tachycardic. On examination, surgical emphysema is present in the suprasternal notch and a chest X-ray shows a pneumomediastinum. What is the most likely diagnosis?

a. Oesophageal perforation.
b. Foreign body ingestion.
c. Oesophageal stricture.
d. Duodenal perforation.

14) A 36-year-old male presents to his primary care doctor with a 4-week history of dysphagia and a sore throat. He has felt fatigued during this period and his friends believe he appears paler than usual. On examination, glossitis, angular stomatitis and koilonychia are present, and bloods reveal a microcytic anaemia. What is the underlying diagnosis?

a. Foreign body.
b. Gastro-oesophageal reflux disease.
c. Plummer-Vinson syndrome.
d. Squamous cell carcinoma.

15) A 32-year-old male presents to the emergency department with abdominal pain and vomiting. On examination, the patient has visible jaundice and is tender in the right upper quadrant and an abdominal ultrasound confirms an extrinsic compression of the common bile duct by a solitary gallstone. What is the most likely diagnosis?

a. Mirizzi syndrome.
b. Choledochal cyst.
c. Ascending cholangitis.
d. Acute pancreatitis.

16) A 35-year-old female undergoes an emergency laparotomy for a perforated posterior duodenal ulcer which has resulted in torrential bleeding. During the laparotomy the ulcer is located in the first part of the duodenum. The consultant asks his medical student using his knowledge of anatomy — which artery is the most likely to be causing the haemorrhage?

a. Superior mesenteric artery.
b. Inferior mesenteric artery.
c. Gastroduodenal artery.
d. Superior pancreaticoduodenal artery.

17) A 45-year-old male is admitted to the emergency department with sudden-onset severe epigastric pain and non-productive retching. An experienced nurse attempts to pass a nasogastric tube without success. A chest X-ray shows a retrocardiac gas-filled viscus with a double air-fluid level. What is the most likely diagnosis?

a. Crohn's disease.
b. Gastric volvulus.
c. Gastric adenocarcinoma.
d. Hiatus hernia.

18) A 52-year-old male is seen in the surgical outpatient clinic following a 12-month history of dysphagia. He has noted a burning sensation and discomfort in his chest following eating which is relieved by belching. Examination is difficult due to obesity but the doctor reviewing the patient believes he can hear bowels sounds in the thoracic cavity. A chest X-ray is ordered which shows a gas bubble and fluid level behind the heart. What is the most likely diagnosis?

a. Sliding hiatus hernia.
b. Rolling hiatus hernia.
c. Gastric volvulus.
d. Erosive gastritis.

19) What is the preferred treatment option for a patient diagnosed with an oesophageal carcinoma that is amenable to surgery in the middle to lower third of the oesophagus?

a.   Right thoracolaparotomy.
b.   Ivor-Lewis procedure.
c.   Left thoracolaparotomy.
d.   Transhiatal approach.

20) A 34-year-old psychiatric patient is reviewed on the surgical assessment unit following a 4-day history of abdominal pain, vomiting and lack of appetite. She has a habitual habit of chewing and eating her own hair. The admitting doctor believes she has a bezoar. What type of bezoar is this patient likely to have?

a.   Small bowel obstruction.
b.   Phytobezoar.
c.   Lactobezoar.
d.   Trichobezoar.

21) A 4-week-old infant is brought to the paediatric emergency department by his family following a 2-day history of non-bilious projectile vomiting which occurred after feeding. The symptoms have been worsening over the past 24 hours and the infant is now lethargic. On examination, he is dehydrated with an olive mass palpable in the epigastrium and peristalsis is evident. What is the underlying diagnosis?

a.   Pyloric stenosis.
b.   Duodenal atresia.
c.   Biliary atresia.
d.   Tracheo-oesophageal fistula.

22) A 45-year-old male presents to the surgical assessment unit with a 48-hour history of fever and abdominal pain. He has recently been treated for acute cholecystitis. On this admission, he has a swinging pyrexia and abdominal examination reveals right upper quadrant tenderness and clinical jaundice. What is the underlying diagnosis?

a. Cholelithiasis.
b. Acute cholecystitis.
c. Liver abscess.
d. Hepatocellular carcinoma.

23) A 2-month-old infant presents to the paediatric surgical clinic with persistent jaundice. He is otherwise fit and well. His parents have noted that his stools are pale and his urine is dark. Ultrasound shows obliterated bile ducts and a shrunken gallbladder. What is the most likely diagnosis?

a. Hydatid cyst.
b. Biliary atresia.
c. Duodenal atresia.
d. Choledochal cyst.

Extended matching questions

Upper gastrointestinal bleeding

a. Oesophageal varices.

b. Gastric ulcer.

c. Duodenal ulcer.

d. Mallory-Weiss tear.

e. Aorto-enteric fistula.

f. Gastric angiodysplasia.

g. Erosive gastritis.

h. Gastric adenocarcinoma.

Match the description with the most likely underlying pathology.

1) A 21-year-old student presents to the emergency department with a 24-hour history of vomiting. He has noticed his last two episodes have contained fresh, bright red blood. The student has been vomiting forcibly for the past 6 hours following an alcohol binge to celebrate his birthday with friends.

2) A 43-year-old male presents to the surgical assessment unit following two episodes of haematemesis at home. He describes the vomit as coffee ground. He has had a dull epigastric pain for the past 6 weeks and pain is worsened by food.

3) A 46-year-old alcoholic patient presents to the emergency department with multiple episodes of haematemesis. On examination, he is jaundiced with spider naevi, hepatomegaly and gross ascites.

4) A 69-year-old female presents to the emergency department with a 24-hour history of severe haematemesis and malaena. She had an endovascular repair of an AAA 6 months ago. On examination, she is tachycardic and hypotensive.

5) A 62-year-old female is referred to the outpatient surgical clinic with a 4-month history of epigastric pain, weight loss and early satiety. She has a history of pernicious anaemia. On examination, she has an epigastric mass and a hard enlarged lymph node in the left supraclavicular fossa.

Hepatopancreatobiliary pathology

a. Acute pancreatitis.   e. Choledochal cyst.
b. Chronic pancreatitis.   f. Ascending cholangitis.
c. Biliary colic.   g. Liver abscess.
d. Acute cholecystitis.   h. Hepatocellular carcinoma.

Match the description of the patient with the most likely diagnosis.

6) A 42-year-old male presents to the emergency department with epigastric pain radiating to the back which started 24 hours ago and is severe in nature. The patient admits to drinking 12 pints of lager per day for the past 6 months and has never had pain like this before. On examination, he has epigastric tenderness.

7) A 38-year-old lady presents to her primary care doctor as a same-day appointment with severe epigastric pain that occurred after eating at a fast food restaurant. She admits to nausea but no vomiting. On examination, she has mild right upper quadrant tenderness. Blood results are unremarkable.

8) A 16-month-old infant undergoes an ultrasound assessment following a prolonged period of jaundice and cholestasis. Ultrasound examination shows a saccular dilation of the common bile duct but normal intrahepatic ducts.

9) A 42-year-old female is admitted to the surgical assessment unit with a 24-hour history of right upper quadrant pain, fever and jaundice. She has a history of gallstones. She has an abdominal ultrasound revealing multiple gallstones in the gallbladder and a dilated common bile duct.

10) A 32-year-old male presents to the emergency department with right upper quadrant pain, lethargy and fever. He has recently travelled to Asia. Observations show he is tachycardic with a swinging pyrexia. Blood results show a raised WCC and CRP. LFTs were unremarkable. Stool cultures are positive for *Entamoeba histolytica*.

Small bowel malignancy

a.	Adenoma.	e.	Lipoma.
b.	Gastrointestinal stromal tumours.	f.	Carcinoid.
c.	Squamous cell carcinoma.	g.	Cholangiocarcinoma.
d.	Lymphoma.	h.	Peutz-Jeghers syndrome.

Match the description of the patient with the most likely diagnosis.

11) This is characterised by multiple intestinal polyps and mucosal melanin spots.

12) This tumour is the most common in the appendix and terminal ileum.

13) These tumours occur commonly in the ileum.

14) This tumour is associated with familial adenomatous polyposis (FAP).

15) These tumours are associated with mutations in c-KIT.

Biliary tract disease

a.	Antibiotics only.	e.	Antibiotics and elective cholecystectomy.
b.	No treatment.	f.	Open cholecystectomy.
c.	MRCP.	g.	Laparoscopic cholecystectomy.
d.	ERCP.	h.	Percutaneous drainage.

Match the description with the most appropriate management option.

16) A 34-year-old male presents to the emergency department with right upper quadrant pain, lethargy and fever. He was discharged 2 days ago with oral antibiotics for acute cholecystitis. Observations show a tachycardia and swinging pyrexia. Blood results show a raised WCC and CRP. LFTs are unremarkable.

17) A 56-year-old male is admitted to the surgical assessment unit with a 36-hour history of right upper quadrant pain and vomiting. The pain is worse following food and he has been unable to eat anything for 24 hours. On examination, he has right upper quadrant tenderness. Blood results show a raised WCC and CRP. The clerking doctor diagnoses the patient with acute cholecystitis.

18) A 45-year-old male presents to the emergency department with a 2-day history of jaundice, nausea and abdominal pain. On examination, he has right upper quadrant pain. He has had previous episodes of pain but not jaundice. An ultrasound of the abdomen shows a dilated common bile duct and solitary gallstone in the common bile duct.

19) A 56-year-old male is admitted with right upper quadrant pain and fever. He is treated for acute cholecystitis with antibiotics but symptoms still persist. What should be arranged to occur within 1 week of admission?

20) A 42-year-old female is admitted to the surgical assessment unit with a 24-hour history of right upper quadrant pain, fever and jaundice. She has a history of gallstones. She has an abdominal ultrasound revealing multiple gallstones in the gallbladder and a dilated common bile duct.

Complications of pancreatitis

a.   ARDS.

b.   Pancreatic pseudocyst.

c.   Pancreatic abscess.

d.   Pseudoaneurysm.

e.   Phlegmon.

f.   Sterile pancreatic necrosis.

g.   Infected pancreatic necrosis.

h.   Exocrine pancreatic insufficiency.

Match the description with the most likely complication of pancreatitis.

21) A 57-year-old male presents to the emergency department with malaena. He is known to have chronic pancreatitis. He had a recent admission for an attack of pancreatitis.

22) A 34-year-old male is admitted to the surgical ward for treatment of acute pancreatitis. Four days into his admission he develops shortness of breath and hypoxia. A chest X-ray reveals bilateral pulmonary opacities and non-cardiogenic pulmonary oedema.

23) A 26-year-old male with chronic pancreatitis attends the general surgery clinic for his regular follow-up. He has noted several episodes of steatorrhoea, weight loss and fatigue. The consultant reviewing the patient decides to commence Creon®.

24) A 40-year-old male is reviewed in the outpatient surgical clinic following admission for acute pancreatitis secondary to gallstones. He informs you that he still has abdominal pain following discharge which is epigastric in nature radiating to the back. Bloods demonstrate a serum amylase of 3400IU/L. On examination, he is tender in the epigastrium but observations are unremarkable.

25) A 42-year-old female is on a surgical ward recovering from acute pancreatitis. She is reviewed on the ward round by the consultant who is concerned regarding her slow recovery. She has a fever and blood tests show a persistently raised WCC. A CT scan shows a region of non-viable pancreatic tissue with air in this area.

Gastric surgical procedures

a.	Billroth I.	e.	Vagotomy, pyloroplasty.
b.	Billroth II.	f.	Roux-en-Y.
c.	Truncal vagotomy.	g.	Selective vagotomy.
d.	Highly selective vagotomy.	h.	Vagotomy, antrectomy, Roux-en-Y.

Match the surgical procedure with the most appropriate indication.

26) This procedure aims to preserve the nerve of Latarjet and remove only the stimulation to the parietal cells in the body of the stomach.

27) This procedure involves the removal of the distal third of the stomach and anastomosis to the duodenum.

28) This procedure can be used as a weight loss surgery and involves a pouch from the greater curvature of the stomach and connecting this directly to the small intestine. The remaining portion of the stomach remains in continuity with the bowel for gastric and digestive secretions.

29) This procedure involves cutting the vagal supply to the stomach resulting in reduced gastric acid secretion and gastric paralysis.

30) This procedure involves the removal of the distal two thirds of the stomach and anastomosis of the greater curvature to the jejunum.

Oesophageal pathology

a.	Achalasia.	e.	Adenocarcinoma.
b.	Oesophageal perforation.	f.	Squamous cell carcinoma.
c.	Oesophageal stricture.	g.	Foreign body.
d.	Barrett's oesophagus.	h.	Globus hystericus.

Match the description of the patient with the most likely diagnosis.

31) A 62-year-old male presents with a 4-month history of progressive dysphagia to solids and recently to liquids. He is currently a smoker. He has noticed a 2-stone unintentional weight loss over the past 4 months. A barium swallow shows a tumour in the lower third of the oesophagus.

32) A 45-year-old male is admitted to the emergency department by ambulance with a sudden-onset pain in his chest, neck and upper abdomen whilst playing in the garden with his nephew. He is hypotensive and tachycardic. A chest X-ray shows the presence of a pneumomediastinum.

33) A 40-year-old female is referred to the surgical outpatient clinic with a 3-month history of dysphagia. Symptoms occur with both solids and liquids. A barium swallow demonstrates oesophageal dilatation and a bird's beak appearance in the distal oesophagus.

34) A 53-year-old male presents with a 6-month history of progressive dysphagia to solids and liquids. He is an ex-smoker who smoked 20 cigarettes per day for 40 years. He believes he has lost weight over the past 4 months. A barium swallow shows a tumour in the middle third of the oesophagus.

35) A 58-year-old male with a prolonged history of gastro-oesophageal reflux disease presents to the outpatient clinic with a 2-month history of dysphagia. A barium swallow confirms the diagnosis.

Upper gastrointestinal malignancy

a. Carcinoid.
b. Peutz-Jeghers syndrome.
c. Gastrointestinal stromal tumour.
d. Lymphoma.
e. Leiomyomas.
f. Adenocarcinoma.
g. Squamous cell carcinoma.
h. Cholangiocarcinoma.

Match the description of the patient with the most likely diagnosis.

36) A 57-year-old male presents to the outpatient clinic with a 12-week history of abdominal pain, nausea, vomiting and diarrhoea. He has noticed a 2-stone unintentional weight loss and on examination he has a flushed appearance. Blood results show a raised serotonin level.

37) A 56-year-old female presents to the surgical outpatient clinic with an 8-week history of dysphagia which has progressed from solids to liquids. She has lost 2 stone in weight over the past 3 months. She has a past medical history of achalasia. On examination, she has cervical lymphadenopathy.

38) A 56-year-old male prevents with a prolonged history of vague abdominal pain and pallor. Blood tests reveal an anaemia. He undergoes an OGD which shows a tumour at the greater curve of the stomach; this undergoes histological analysis revealing a c-KIT gene mutation.

39) A 23-year-old female is admitted to the surgical assessment unit with abdominal pain and failure to pass flatus for 24 hours. Examination notes the presence of hamartomatous polyps causing an intussusception. She is also noted to have multiple areas of mucocutaneous pigmentation.

40) An 82-year-old male presents to the surgical outpatient clinic with a 12-week history of dysphagia which has progressed from solids to liquids. He has lost 3 stone in weight over the past 4 months. He has a past medical history of Barrett's oesophagus. On examination, he has cervical lymphadenopathy.

Splenic pathology

a. Hyposplenism.
b. Hypersplenism.
c. Splenic abscess.
d. Trauma.

e. Portal vein thrombosis.
f. Laparoscopic splenectomy.
g. Thrombocytosis.
h. Open splenectomy.

Match the description of the patient with the most appropriate option.

41) A 23-year-old male undergoes an emergency splenectomy following a car accident. Following the procedure he asks what is the most common complication following a splenectomy.

42) A 23-year-old male with a previous history of bacterial endocarditis is listed for an elective splenectomy due to progressive splenomegaly. He has had a swinging pyrexia and left upper quadrant pain. On examination, there is mild oedema of the soft tissues overlying the spleen.

43) A 29-year-old female with coeliac disease has a blood film performed which shows Howell-Jolly bodies and Pappenheimer bodies.

44) A 56-year-old male with idiopathic thrombocytopenic purpura is reviewed in the general surgery clinic following the failure of medical treatment to control his condition. On examination, the patient has multiple petechiae but no organomegaly is felt. The junior doctor asks his consultant what would be the best approach for this operation.

45) A 45-year-old male is listed for an elective splenectomy following a 6-month history of anaemia, thrombocytopaenia and leucopenia.

Short answer questions

1) A 32-year-old female presents to the emergency department with right upper quadrant pain and jaundice for 24 hours. On examination, she is pyrexial at 38.7°C, tachycardic and jaundiced.

a.	Define Charcot's triad.	3 marks
b.	What is cholangitis?	1 mark
c.	Give two causes of cholangitis.	1 mark
d.	Name three potential complications of obstructive jaundice.	3 marks
e.	Which bacteria are these patients susceptible to and why?	2 marks

2) A 26-year-old female presents to the emergency department with a 6-hour history of right upper quadrant pain. She describes the pain as colicky in nature and often follows ingestion of food. You are concerned about gallstones.

a.	What are gallstones made of?	2 marks
b.	Describe the metabolism of bilirubin.	3 marks
c.	What is the gold standard investigation for gallstones?	1 mark
d.	She is found to have a common bile duct obstructing calculus. What are her treatment options?	3 marks
e.	Name two other complications of gallstone disease that would lead to the patient needing a cholecystectomy sooner than 18 weeks.	1 mark

3) A 63-year-old male visits his primary care doctor with a 9-month history of dyspepsia following meals. He has tried several home treatments with no effect.

a. State three lifestyle advice options which may improve symptoms. 3 marks
b. Define Barrett's oesophagus. 2 marks
c. Name the two types of oesophageal cancer. 2 marks
d. State the two most common causes of squamous cell carcinoma. 2 marks
e. A patient with metastatic oesophageal cancer is admitted with recurrent vomiting. What treatment could you consider? 1 mark

4) A 53-year-old male presents to the emergency department with an 18-hour history of severe epigastric pain radiating to the back. He has a past medical history of excessive alcohol use. On examination, he is tender in the epigastrium and blood results show an amylase of 4300IU/L.

a. What is the underlying diagnosis? 1 mark
b. Name three immediate actions that could be performed. 3 marks
c. Specify the scoring system commonly used in this condition. 1 mark
d. State three additional treatments that may be required. 3 marks
e. Give two complications of this condition. 2 marks

5) A 24-year-old male is reviewed in the emergency department by the on-call general surgery doctor, who lists the patient for an urgent splenectomy.

a. Name three indications for a splenectomy. 3 marks
b. Specify two prophylactic measures following a splenectomy. 2 marks
c. List three bacteria post-splenectomy patients are susceptible to. 3 marks
d. What complication is caused by the above bacteria? 1 mark
e. What is a splenunculus? 1 mark

6) A 52-year-old male presents to his primary care doctor with a 6-week history of epigastric pain, which is worse on eating. He does not take any medication. The primary care doctor is concerned about a diagnosis of peptic ulcer disease.

a.	Define four causes of peptic ulcer disease.	2 marks
b.	List three differences between gastric and duodenal ulcers.	3 marks
c.	State the gold standard investigation for peptic ulcer disease.	1 mark
d.	Name one complication of peptic ulcer disease.	1 mark
e.	State three management options for peptic ulcer disease.	3 marks

7) An 88-year-old female presents to her primary care doctor with a 3-month history of epigastric pain, weight loss and early satiety. She was previously treated for a *H. pylori* infection 10 years ago. On examination, she has epigastric pain and an enlarged lymph node in the left supraclavicular fossa.

a.	What is the underlying diagnosis?	1 mark
b.	Define Troisier's sign and what does this indicate?	1 mark
c.	Specify four predisposing factors relating to gastric cancer.	4 marks
d.	What is TNM staging?	3 marks
e.	Name one method to stage a tumour.	1 mark

8) A 26-year-old male with chronic pancreatitis attends the general surgery clinic for his regular follow-up. He has noted several episodes of steatorrhoea, weight loss and fatigue.

a.	Name two other symptoms of chronic pancreatitis.	2 marks
b.	Specify two investigations for these patients.	2 marks
c.	What may be shown on imaging?	1 mark
d.	Give four long-term treatment options for this patient.	4 marks
e.	What team may be useful in helping to manage this patient?	1 mark

9) A 39-year-old obese female attends her primary care doctor with a 6-month history of intermittent dysphagia. She has noted a burning sensation and discomfort in her chest following eating which is relieved by belching. A chest X-ray shows a gas bubble and fluid level behind the heart.

a.	Name two risk factors for this condition.	1 mark
b.	Define the two main types of hiatus hernia.	2 marks
c.	Specify two clinical features for each type of hiatus hernia.	4 marks
d.	Give two treatment options for this patient.	2 marks
e.	Give two complications of this condition.	1 mark

10) A 42-year-old female presents to the emergency department with a 48-hour history of vomiting and abdominal pain. She has noted abdominal distention and in the last 24 hours has not opened her bowels or passed any flatus. On examination, she has a distended abdomen and auscultation reveals tinkling bowel sounds. An abdominal X-ray shows central, dilated loops of bowel with valvulae conniventes present on these loops.

a.	What is the underlying diagnosis?	1 mark
b.	State three causes for this condition.	3 marks
c.	Give two medical treatments for this patient.	2 marks
d.	If medical treatment fails, how should she be managed?	2 marks
e.	Name two complications of this condition.	2 marks

11) A 72-year-old female with primary sclerosing cholangitis presents to the outpatient clinic with a 3-month history of weight loss and jaundice. On examination, she has abdominal distention, shifting dullness and right upper quadrant abdominal pain. Bloods reveal an elevated α-fetoprotein.

a.	What is the most common primary liver tumour?	1 mark
b.	Which tumour marker is often raised in this condition?	1 mark
c.	Specify four risk factors for this condition.	4 marks
d.	Name two investigations to diagnose this condition.	2 marks
e.	State two treatment options for this patient.	2 marks

12) A 56-year-old male presents with a 5-month history of painless jaundice, anorexia and weight loss. He has noted pale stools and dark urine for the past 3 months. On examination, the gallbladder is palpable but non-tender. He has multiple transient swellings and redness of limb veins. Blood results show a raised CA19-9.

a.	Name four causes of obstructive jaundice.	4 marks
b.	What is the most likely diagnosis in this patient?	2 marks
c.	What should be done prior to commencing any treatment?	1 mark
d.	Name two surgical procedures that may be performed.	2 marks
e.	If the tumour was non-operable, name one treatment option.	1 mark

13) A 42-year-old male presents to his primary care doctor with a 6-month history of dyspepsia and epigastric pain following food. He has noticed he has a dry cough in the morning. He denies any weight loss. The doctor suspects he has gastro-oesophageal reflux disease and commences a first-line therapy.

a. What is the underlying diagnosis?   1 mark
b. Specify four precipitating factors for this condition.   4 marks
c. Give two other symptoms the patient may experience.   2 marks
d. State two investigations that can be arranged for this patient.   2 marks
e. Name one complication of this condition.   1 mark

Chapter 2

Lower GI surgery
QUESTIONS

Single best answer questions

1) Which of these is a complication of Meckel's diverticulum?

a. *Clostridium difficile* infection.
b. Gastrointestinal bleeding.
c. Overgrowth of *Escherichia coli*.
d. Small bowel carcinoma.

2) What is the correct first-line antibiotic for uncomplicated *Clostridium difficile* infection?

a. Cefuroxime.
b. Gentamicin.
c. Metronidazole.
d. Vancomycin.

3) What is the blood supply to the hepatic flexure?

a. Hepatic artery.
b. Left colic artery.
c. Right colic artery.
d. Right gastric artery.

4) Which of these is not a site of portosystemic anastomosis?

a. Distal oesophagus.
b. Pancreas.
c. Rectum.
d. Umbilicus.

5) Which surgical emergency is most likely to result from ulcerative colitis?

a. Caecal volvulus.
b. Necrotising enterocolitis.
c. Perforated Meckel's diverticulum.
d. Toxic megacolon.

6) What is the point of division between the midgut and the hindgut?

a. Caecum.
b. One third of the way along the transverse colon.
c. Splenic flexure.
d. Two thirds of the way along the transverse colon.

7) A patient with appendicitis has pain in the right iliac fossa when the left iliac fossa is palpated. What is this sign?

a. Grey-Turner's sign.
b. McBurney's sign.
c. Murphy's sign.
d. Rovsing's sign.

8) Which of these muscles is not included in the pelvic floor?

a. Coccygeus.
b. Internal anal sphincter.
c. Pubococcygeus.
d. Puborectalis.

9) Which of these is an osmotic laxative?

a. Ispaghula husk.
b. Lactulose.
c. Senna.
d. Sodium docusate.

10) A female patient weighing 82kg has a serum potassium of 4.2mmol/L. She is a Type 2 diabetic and is not on insulin. She has been noted as nil by mouth. Which of these maintenance fluid regimes would be most appropriate for the next 24 hours?

a. 1L 0.9% sodium chloride, 1.5L 5% dextrose, 60mmol potassium.
b. 2.5L Hartmann's solution.
c. 2.5L Hartmann's solution with 60mmol potassium.
d. 2.5L 0.9% sodium chloride, 60mmol potassium.

11) Which of these antibiotics has the highest risk of causing *Clostridium difficile* infection?

a. Ciprofloxacin.
b. Levofloxacin.
c. Moxifloxacin.
d. Ofloxacin.

12) Which of these is not a risk factor for symptomatic haemorrhoids?

a. Constipation.
b. Diarrhoea.
c. Extended sitting.
d. Multiparity.

13) A 76-year-old man has a tumour removed from the transverse colon. On histological examination, the tumour is found to have spread into the muscularis propria. The lymph nodes are free of tumour. What is the stage of this tumour?

a. Dukes A.
b. Dukes B.
c. Dukes C.
d. Dukes D.

14) What is the most appropriate investigation for suspected bowel perforation?

a. Abdominal ultrasound.
b. Abdominal X-ray.
c. Diagnostic laparoscopy.
d. Erect chest X-ray.

15) What is the type of epithelium in the anal canal inferior to the pectinate line?

a. Columnar.
b. Keratinised squamous.
c. Non-keratinised squamous.
d. Stratified.

16) Which of these structures passes through the inguinal canal?

a. Ilio-hypogastric nerve.
b. Ilio-inguinal nerve.
c. Inferior epigastric artery.
d. Pudendal nerve.

17) Which cancer in addition to colorectal cancer is more common in hereditary non-polyposis colon cancer?

a. Breast.
b. Lung.
c. Ovarian.
d. Prostate.

18) You see a patient with a spouted stoma in the right iliac fossa. Which type of stoma is this most likely to be?

a. Colostomy.
b. Ileostomy.
c. Jejunostomy.
d. Urostomy.

19) An operation is performed where the sigmoid colon is removed and a temporary stoma is created. What is the name of this operation?

a. Abdominoperineal resection.
b. Anterior resection.
c. Hartmann's procedure.
d. Whipple's procedure.

20) Which of these is appropriate medical management of an anal fissure?

a. Topical bisoprolol.
b. Topical glyceryl trinitrate.
c. Topical isosorbide mononitrate.
d. Topical verapamil.

21) What is the blood supply to the anal canal above the pectinate line?

a. Anal artery.
b. Inferior rectal artery.
c. Internal pudendal artery.
d. Superior rectal artery.

22) What is the most appropriate investigation for suspected diverticulitis?

a. Abdominal X-ray.
b. Abdominal ultrasound.
c. CT of the abdomen.
d. Erect chest X-ray.

23) Which is a feature of ulcerative colitis?

a. Crypt abscesses.
b. Granulomas.
c. Skip lesions.
d. Transmural inflammation.

Extended matching questions

Abdominal X-rays

a. Coffee bean sign.
b. Dilated bowel loops with valvulae conniventes.
c. Dilated bowel loops with haustra.
d. Opaque round objects at the periphery of the abdomen.
e. Rigler's sign.
f. Sentinel loop.
g. Soft tissue dense opacity in rectum.
h. Thumbprinting.

Match the X-ray findings to the the most likely diagnosis.

1) Constipation.

2) Crohn's disease.

3) Sigmoid volvulus.

4) Bowel perforation.

5) Small bowel obstruction.

Rectal bleeding

a. Anal fissure.
b. Caecal carcinoma.
c. Diverticular disease.
d. Haemorrhoids.

e. Radiation proctitis.
f. Rectal carcinoma.
g. Trauma.
h. Ulcerative colitis.

Match the description of the patient with the most likely diagnosis.

6) A 63-year-old male presents with dark red blood on the outside of his stools. He feels tired and his haemoglobin is 88.

7) A 24-year-old female sees her primary care doctor because she has lower abdominal pain. She is feeling generally unwell and has been noticing blood and mucus in her stools for the past 3 days.

8) A 30-year-old chef has been trying the food too often and has to go to a weight loss group. While he is there he sees fresh red blood in the toilet after opening his bowels.

9) A 44-year-old female has extreme pain when opening her bowels and is very worried because she has noticed bright red blood on the toilet paper when wiping. The primary care doctor is unable to do a rectal examination because it is too painful.

10) An 86-year-old male attends the emergency department with fresh red bleeding in between opening his bowels. He does not have any pain and feels otherwise well. He is pleased that he has lost 5kg in the last 2 months.

Change in bowel habit

a.   Caecal volvulus.

b.   *Campylobacter jejuni.*

c.   Drug-induced.

d.   Paralytic ileus.

e.   Rectal carcinoma.

f.   Sigmoid volvulus.

g.   Small bowel obstruction.

h.   Ulcerative colitis.

Match the description of the patient with the most likely diagnosis.

11)   A 52-year-old male has recently returned to the ward from a laparoscopic appendicectomy and seems to be recovering well. After 2 days his bowels have still not opened and he is vomiting.

12)   A 47-year-old female with Down's syndrome is admitted after not having opened her bowels for 1 week. She has abdominal distention. She has come in with the same problem five times before.

13)   A 19-year-old female has had vomiting and diarrhoea for the past 2 days. The symptoms started after a night out. She admits to taking ecstasy recreationally.

14)   An 89-year-old man with metastatic melanoma has suffered abdominal pains for the past 3 days. You are asked to review him as he has been using the maximum dose of his required pain medication during this time. He has not opened his bowels for 5 days.

15)   A 77-year-old female visits her primary care doctor with watery diarrhoea which she has had for a week. Before this she mentions that she was constipated.

Abdominal pain

a. Appendicitis.

b. Constipation.

c. Diabetic ketoacidosis.

d. Diverticulitis.

e. Foreign body.

f. Gastroenteritis.

g. Ovarian cyst rupture.

h. Ulcerative colitis.

Match the description of the patient with the most likely diagnosis.

16) A 58-year-old female has been brought into the emergency department with lower abdominal pain. Her temperature is 38°C. Her chest X-ray shows air under the right hemi-diaphragm.

17) A 27-year-old male returns from the operating theatre after an operation. He has woken and has severe abdominal pain and vomiting. His blood sugars are 16.2mmol/L and ketones are 0.1mmol/L. He has a temperature of 38.2°C.

18) A 19-year-old female has come in with right-sided abdominal tenderness with guarding. She has vomited twice and has not eaten since yesterday.

19) A 42-year-old male has lower abdominal pain and has not passed stool for 3 days. On examination, his abdomen is mostly soft with tenderness in the lower left quadrant and a palpable descending colon.

20) A 24-year-old female has come in with central abdominal pain, profuse vomiting and diarrhoea, and a temperature of 37.1°C. She reports no change in diet recently.

Examination findings

a. Caput medusae.   e. Psoas sign.
b. Cullen's sign.   f. Rebound tenderness.
c. Grey-Turner's sign.   g. Rigler's sign.
d. Murphy's sign.   h. Rovsing's sign.

Match the examination findings with their description.

21) Bruising of both flanks, indicating pancreatitis.

22) Pain on palpation worsened by relieving pressure, indicating peritonitis.

23) Abdominal pain on extending the right hip, indicating appendicitis.

24) Pain on inspiration when palpating below the right costal margin, suggesting cholecystitis.

25) Air visible on both sides of the bowel wall on abdominal X-ray, indicating a pneumoperitoneum.

Abdominal distention

a.	Ascites.	e.	Obesity.
b.	Bowel stricture.	f.	Pregnancy.
c.	Constipation.	g.	Ruptured AAA.
d.	Incarcerated inguinal hernia.	h.	Transverse colon tumour.

Match the description with the most likely diagnosis.

26) A 47-year-old female has had growing abdominal distention over the past few months. She now weighs 27 stone. She has not had a menstrual period in 4 years.

27) A 55-year-old male has sudden, intense abdominal pain and rapidly growing distention. He has marked central obesity and came in for a hernia repair. His blood pressure is low and falling further.

28) An 82-year-old male has been having treatment for prostate cancer. He comes in with abdominal distention. He has not opened his bowels for 3 days, and he has vomited twice.

29) A 69-year-old female has come into hospital with dizziness, shortness of breath and chest pain. She has noticed partially altered blood mixed in with her stool. On examination, there is abdominal distention and a painless mass in the umbilical region.

30) A 56-year-old male with ulcerative colitis attends the emergency department with a markedly distended abdomen. On examination, there is a shifting dullness.

Anorectal problems

a.	Anal fissure.	e.	Perianal abscess.
b.	Anorectal prolapse.	f.	Pilonidal abscess.
c.	Fistula in ano.	g.	Pilonidal sinus.
d.	Haemorrhoids.	h.	Rectal polyp.

Match the description with the most likely diagnosis.

31) A 65-year-old female with COPD sees her primary care doctor because she has noticed a mass protruding after defaecation. She cannot feel the mass the rest of the time. She is very embarrassed because she has had two episodes where she has lost control of her bowels and not got to the toilet in time.

32) A 37-year-old male arrives in the emergency department with an acutely hot and painful lump on his bottom. On examination, there is a 3cm warm, tender, erythematous swelling in the natal cleft, 6cm superior to the anus. The patient says he has had an operation for this problem once before.

33) A 72-year-old female consults her primary care doctor asking for a cream because she has noticed discharge around her anus for the last 2 weeks. This is causing her to have itching and pain. Her past medical history includes osteoporosis, diverticular disease and rheumatoid arthritis.

34) An 8-year-old male is brought to the emergency department by his uncle because he has noticed bright red blood in the toilet after opening his bowels. When the doctor attempts an examination he screams and runs away.

35) A 44-year-old male rushes into the emergency department complaining of severe pain. He says he has not been able to open his bowels for 2 days due to the pain. On examination, he is obese and there is a 3cm warm, tender, erythematous swelling just to the left of the anal verge. His past medical history includes asthma and Type 2 diabetes.

Genetics

a.   Cowden disease.   e.   MEN 1.
b.   Familial adenomatous polyposis.   f.   MYH-associated polyposis.
c.   Lynch syndrome.   g.   Peutz-Jeghers syndrome.
d.   Li-Fraumeni syndrome.   h.   von Hippel-Lindau syndrome.

Match the description of the patient with the most likely genetic problem.

36) A 46-year-old male loses 10kg over 2 months and develops iron deficiency anaemia. On colonoscopy, he is diagnosed with an adenocarcinoma in the ascending colon. Due to his age he is asked about his family history and says that his mother died of endometrial cancer when she was 61 and his older sister has been treated for a rectal tumour. His father is well with no significant health problems.

37) A 29-year-old female has a gastroscopy due to reflux symptoms. She is found to have multiple polyps in the duodenum. She also has brown spots in her mouth. Her father is currently being treated for colon cancer.

38) A 26-year-old male is brought to the resuscitation area following a car crash. On examination, he has an ileostomy. When his family arrive they explain that he has had his colon removed because doctors said he was at increased risk of cancer. Several other family members have had the same operation.

39) A 52-year-old female has a colonoscopy due to rectal bleeding, which shows multiple polyps. She is also noted to have papules on her face, especially around the mouth. She has previously had a mastectomy for breast cancer.

40) A 39-year-old female develops a lump on her thigh and is diagnosed with a rhabdomyosarcoma. When asked about her family history, she says that her father was treated for an osteosarcoma 10 years ago and her younger sister is undergoing follow-up for a colorectal cancer which was resected at age 28 years.

Weight loss

a. Palliative management.
b. Anterior resection.
c. Defunctioning loop colostomy.
d. Hartmann's procedure.

e. Left hemicolectomy.
f. Mesalazine and steroids.
g. Right hemicolectomy.
h. Total colectomy.

Match the description with the most appropriate management.

41) An 87-year-old male sees his primary care doctor because he has lost 15kg over the last 10 weeks. He feels generally unwell and fatigued and bloods show a new iron deficiency anaemia. He is referred to have a colonoscopy which shows a circumferential tumour in the ascending colon. A CT scan reveals metastases to the liver with several peritoneal deposits.

42) A 55-year-old female has lost 6kg in the last month. She has recently noticed some dark streaks of blood on the outside of her stools. She is sent for a colonoscopy which shows a mass in the ascending colon. A biopsy shows that the mass is an adenocarcinoma.

43) A 25-year-old male with ulcerative colitis is admitted under gastroenterology with fever and abdominal pain. He has lost 5kg in the last 2 weeks and has a reduced appetite. His pain increases 2 days into his admission and he has an abdominal X-ray, which shows thumbprinting in loops of bowel around the periphery, and air under both hemidiaphragms.

44) A 75-year-old female visits her primary care doctor after losing 5kg in the past 4 weeks. She says she does not feel like eating. Her visit today has been provoked by an episode of fresh red bleeding after she opened her bowels yesterday. On digital rectal examination, a hard craggy mass is felt.

45) A 46-year-old male doctors' receptionist asks to see one of the doctors as he has developed vomiting and diarrhoea. He is worried because he has felt unable to eat and drink for the last 2 days and has lost 2kg when weighing himself on the practice scales.

Short answer questions

1) A 64-year-old female presents to the emergency department with left-sided abdominal pain and feeling generally unwell. On examination, she is pyrexial and has tenderness in the left iliac fossa. The doctor suspects diverticulitis.

a. State the difference between diverticulosis and diverticulitis. 1 mark
b. What is the best investigation to confirm the diagnosis? 1 mark
c. State four ways this patient may be managed and followed up. 4 marks
d. Name two potential complications of diverticulitis. 2 marks
e. Suggest two aspects of lifestyle advice that she could be given to reduce future episodes. 2 marks

2) A 31-year-old male has had a reversal of an ileostomy 3 days previously and is drinking fluids normally. He has also had some soup. The junior doctor is called to see him because he has vomited three times. He says he is feeling very sick and has not yet opened his bowels or passed flatus since the surgery. On examination, his abdomen is distended. The doctor thinks the patient has developed a postoperative ileus.

a. Define the term 'ileus'. 2 marks
b. What investigation and result may aid the diagnosis? 2 marks
c. What should the doctor do to acutely manage the patient? 2 marks
d. What is the prognosis for this patient? 1 mark
e. Name three causes of a bowel obstruction. 3 marks

3) A 78-year-old male sees his primary care doctor with a history of constipation followed by diarrhoea. He is referred to colorectal surgery urgently due to a concern that his symptoms may be due to malignancy.

a. State which investigation would help confirm the diagnosis. 1 mark

b. If the diagnosis of colorectal cancer is confirmed, what two investigations are needed to decide on treatment? 2 marks

c. Describe how an adenocarcinoma develops in the colon. 4 marks

d. What screening programs are in place in the UK for bowel cancer and how do they work? 2 marks

e. This patient's tumour is at the splenic flexure. Which operation is most appropriate to safely remove it? 1 mark

4) A 24-year-old male sees his primary care doctor because he has been experiencing bleeding when opening his bowels. The blood is bright red and he notices it on the toilet paper or in the toilet, but not mixed in with his stools. He is otherwise well. The doctor diagnoses haemorrhoids.

a. Name two risk factors for developing haemorrhoids. 2 marks

b. State the difference between internal and external haemorrhoids. 1 mark

c. Name two other causes for fresh rectal bleeding. 2 marks

d. How might the primary care doctor treat this problem? 2 marks

e. State three options for management if this treatment fails. 3 marks

5) A 47-year-old female has previously had an open right hemicolectomy for an ascending colon carcinoma. She has recovered well and has not had any signs of disease recurrence on follow-up. However, she develops a bulging in the lower part of her laparotomy scar. Her primary care doctor examines her and finds an incisional hernia.

a. State two features that should be assessed on examination. 2 marks
b. Describe how an incisional hernia is formed. 2 marks
c. Name three risk factors for developing an incisional hernia. 3 marks
d. State how this patient should be managed. 1 mark
e. Give two complications that may result from this condition. 2 marks

6) An 8-year-old boy is brought to the emergency department with abdominal pain. He says that the pain started 2 days ago in the centre of his abdomen but has now moved to the right lower quadrant. On examination, he is tender in the right iliac fossa and his temperature is 38.6°C.

a. Give two other findings suggestive of an acute appendicitis. 2 marks
b. Describe how appendicitis may develop. 2 marks
c. How should this patient be managed? 1 mark
d. Name two other causes of pain in the right iliac fossa. 2 marks
e. On examination, the patient also has a palpable mass in the right iliac fossa. What complication of appendicitis does this suggest and how should it be treated? 3 marks

7) A 29-year-old male is seen by an out-of-hours primary care doctor because he has developed a painful red swelling between his buttocks. He has had this problem once before 2 years ago and was treated in hospital. The doctor suspects a pilonidal abscess.

a. What is a pilonidal sinus and how does this lead to a pilonidal abscess? — 3 marks

b. What medical treatment might the primary care doctor offer? — 1 mark

c. The patient returns as the abscess has got larger. What management is needed now? — 1 mark

d. Name three risk factors for pilonidal sinus disease. — 3 marks

e. State two ways to reduce the likelihood of future abscesses. — 2 marks

8) A 20-year-old female arrives at the emergency department as she is feeling unwell. She has been having bloody diarrhoea up to six times a day and has abdominal pain. On examination, she is tachycardic and her temperature is 38.1°C. She has a known diagnosis of ulcerative colitis and is taking mesalazine.

a. Name two pathological features of ulcerative colitis. — 2 marks

b. State two features that might be seen on an abdominal X-ray. — 2 marks

c. How would it be decided if she needs an operation? — 2 marks

d. Name two extra gastrointestinal features of ulcerative colitis. — 2 marks

e. Suggest two complications in a flare of ulcerative colitis. — 2 marks

9) A 57-year-old male has had an open inguinal hernia repair. Two days after the operation his wound dressing is changed and the nurses call the doctor to see the patient because they are concerned he has a wound infection.

a. State two wound findings that would suggest an infection.   2 marks

b. List two precautions that should be taken in theatre to prevent   2 marks
    surgical site infection.

c. Name three risk factors for postoperative wound infection.   3 marks

d. Name one investigation to assess the severity of infection.   1 mark

e. Give two methods to treat this patient.   2 marks

10) A 91-year-old male has a defunctioning ileostomy because
    he has small bowel obstruction due to an ascending colon
    tumour.

a. State two examination features to suggest it is an ileostomy.   2 marks

b. Name two other types of stoma.   2 marks

c. The patient develops high output from his stoma. State two ways to 2 marks
    manage this complication.

d. Name two other potential complications of a stoma.   2 marks

e. Describe two features when examining a stoma that would suggest it 2 marks
    is not healthy and functioning normally.

11) A 21-year-old female with a history of self-harm is brought
    to the emergency department by her partner because she
    has swallowed several nails. She is complaining of
    abdominal pain and is tachycardic and pyrexial, so doctors
    are concerned she may have a bowel perforation.

a. State two features on examination to suggest a perforation.   2 marks

b. Name three other causes of gastrointestinal tract perforation.   3 marks

c. What investigation may support the diagnosis?   1 mark

d. State two methods for managing this.   2 marks

e. List two sites where foreign bodies are likely to be impacted.   2 marks

12) A 53-year-old male is seen by his primary care doctor with sudden-onset abdominal pain, nausea and vomiting. His history includes hypertension, angina and he is morbidly obese. He has not passed stool since the pain started 1 hour ago. The doctor is concerned about ischaemic colitis.

a. Name four other risk factors for ischaemic colitis.   4 marks
b. Which parts of the bowel are most likely to be affected?   1 mark
c. This man's superior mesenteric artery has become occluded. Which   2 marks
    sections of his bowel have been affected?
d. What is the most appropriate management for this patient?   2 marks
e. If the patient does not improve with initial treatment and no cause   1 mark
    has yet been identified, what is the next step in management?

13) A 52-year-old male is seen in the emergency department as he has abdominal distention and pain. He has not opened his bowels for 7 days and today he has started vomiting. After performing an abdominal X-ray, doctors diagnose that his symptoms are caused by a volvulus.

a. What is a volvulus?   1 mark
b. What part of the bowel is most likely to be affected and what would   2 marks
    its appearance be on the X-ray?
c. Name two risk factors for a volvulus.   2 marks
d. State one method to manage this patient and two features that   3 marks
    suggest surgical management is indicated.
e. Name two complications of a volvulus.   2 marks

Chapter 3

Vascular surgery
QUESTIONS

1) A 65-year-old male presents to the emergency department with a 3-hour history of severe central abdominal and lower back pain which started all of a sudden. On examination, he is found to be pale, hypotensive, tachycardic and has a prolonged capillary refill time at 5 seconds. Further examination notes the absence of a right femoral pulse. What is the most likely diagnosis?

a. Aortic dissection.
b. Mesenteric ischaemia.
c. Ruptured AAA.
d. Acute limb ischaemia.

2) A 56-year-old female attends her primary care doctor with a painless wound on her left leg which has been present for 6 weeks. On examination, you note a 2 x 3cm ulcer on the medial malleolus which is irregular in shape. Further inspection of the wound reveals it is shallow with a base of granulation tissue. Skin temperature is normal and pulses and skin sensation are intact. What is the most likely diagnosis?

a. Arterial ulcer.
b. Venous ulcer.
c. Neuropathic ulcer.
d. Traumatic ulcer.

3) A 22-year-old female presents to the emergency department with sudden-onset pain and swelling in her left leg. On examination, she is tender in her left calf and it is 4cm larger than the right; it feels warm and superficial veins are engorged. On passive dorsiflexion of the foot, she experiences pain in her calf. Pulses are present and the rest of her examination is normal. What is the underlying diagnosis?

a. Cellulitis.
b. Deep vein thrombosis.
c. Acute limb ischaemia.
d. Ruptured popliteal aneurysm.

4) A 68-year-old male presents to his primary care doctor with a 2-week history of pain in his right leg; the pain has been severe and he has used Oramorph® with little effect. He is experiencing the worst pain at night; however, it still occurs during the day even at rest. On examination,

several arterial ulcers are noted and there is reduced sensation in the right foot. What is the most likely diagnosis?

a. Intermittent claudication.
b. Acute limb ischaemia.
c. Critical limb ischaemia.
d. Raynaud's syndrome.

5) A 58-year-old female presents to the vascular clinic with a painful wound on her right leg which has been present for the past 4 weeks. The wound is on the forefoot and is well demarcated with a regular shape which appears to be punched out. No granulation tissue is present and the underlying ligament is visible; skin sensation is intact but pulses are absent. What is the most likely diagnosis?

a. Arterial ulcer.
b. Venous ulcer.
c. Neuropathic ulcer.
d. Traumatic ulcer.

6) A 60-year-old male smoker attends his primary care doctor with pain in his right left leg which feels like a muscle cramp following walking for short distances; he has noted that he can now walk 500m before he gets pain in his leg when previously this was up to a mile. He experiences pain in his right calf but does not experience chest pain or shortness of breath. What is the most likely diagnosis?

a. Intermittent claudication.
b. Critical limb ischaemia.
c. Sciatica.
d. Leriche's syndrome.

7) A 76-year-old female presents to her primary care doctor as she has noticed an itchy and scaly area around her ankles with an associated rash; she is known to have varicose veins. On examination, you note a pale red rash which is not painful to the touch and the skin appears flaky. What complication related to her varicose veins has this patient developed?

a. Haemorrhage.
b. Thrombophlebitis.
c. Lipodermatosclerosis.
d. Venous eczema.

8) A 26-year-old female presents to her primary care doctor with two episodes of her fingers changing colour in the cold weather. She has no other symptoms. She explains that her fingers go initially white, then blue, and finally red before returning to their normal colour during cold weather. Examination is normal. What is the most likely diagnosis?

a. Takayasu's arteritis.
b. Buerger's disease.
c. Subclavian steal syndrome.
d. Raynaud's syndrome.

9) A 34-year-old male attends his primary care doctor with a painful and swollen right arm which occurs mainly after strenuous activity. He has noted his right hand appears to be colder and weaker than the left. On examination, the symptoms are made worse by raising the patient's arm above his head with opening and closing of the fist. Wasting of the small muscles of the hand are noted. What is the most likely diagnosis?

a. Renal artery stenosis.
b. Vascular malformation.
c. Thoracic outlet syndrome.
d. Subclavian steal syndrome.

10) A 76-year-old female Type 2 diabetic attends the diabetic clinic for regular review. On examination of her feet, you notice a disorganised arrangement of the bone structure and loss of sensation around the joint. The foot has a limited range of motion and is swollen. What is the underlying diagnosis?

a. Charcot joint.
b. Neuropathic ulcer.
c. Pyoderma gangrenosum.
d. Arterial ulcer.

11) A 70-year-old male presents to the emergency department with a severely painful right limb for the past 4 hours. He has a past medical history of peripheral vascular disease. He has not been able to move his leg for the past 2 hours. On examination, he has an absent capillary refill, paralysis and loss of sensation in the right leg. Arterial and venous Doppler are unable to locate a signal. What is the most appropriate treatment for this patient?

a. Angioplasty.
b. Embolectomy.
c. Amputation.
d. Thrombolysis.

12) You are the junior doctor on-call for the vascular surgery ward at a large teaching hospital. The ward contacts you to urgently review a 68-year-old female who underwent a right angioplasty procedure 24 hours ago for acute limb ischaemia. Her right leg is painful and her observations show she is tachycardic, tachypnoeic, hypotensive and her most recent bloods show acute renal failure which was not present on admission. What is the most likely diagnosis?

a. Renal artery stenosis.
b. Reperfusion injury.
c. Compartment syndrome.
d. Haemorrhage.

13) A 78-year-old male attends the vascular surgery clinic following a TIA 7 days ago. He undergoes a duplex ultrasound which shows a stenosis of 78% in his right internal carotid artery. What is the most appropriate treatment for this patient?

a. Coronary artery bypass grafting.
b. Ankle-brachial pulse index.
c. Carotid endarterectomy.
d. Anticoagulation only.

14) A 67-year-old female presents to the vascular clinic with a history of buttock and thigh pain for the past 6 weeks. The consultant in charge of her care believes her disease lies at the level of the common iliac artery. What would the

difference be if the disease was due to stenosis at the aorto-iliac junction?

a. Pulses would be lost bilaterally.
b. Symptoms would only affect the calf.
c. Only the buttock and thigh would be involved.
d. ABPI would be normal.

15) A 70-year-old male is admitted to the emergency department with a suspected aortic dissection. What type of dissection would this patient have if he was to undergo urgent surgery rather than initial medical management?

a. Stanford Type A.
b. Stanford Type B.
c. Fontaine II.
d. De Bakey III.

16) Which of the following is a feature of critical limb ischaemia?

a. Pain at rest.
b. Pain on exercise relieved when stopping.
c. Ankle systolic pressure >50mmHg.
d. Pain relieved by simple analgesia.

17) A 76-year-old female attends her primary care doctor with increasing pain in her right leg following a period of exercise. She can walk 400m before she has pain in her right calf which is relieved on stopping and simple analgesia. She has a past medical history of hypertension and is an ex-smoker. On examination, she has a cool and pale lower limb with weak peripheral pulses. An ABPI examination is performed. What would you expect the result to be in this patient?

a.   >1
b.   0.8
c.   0.6
d.   0.4

18) A 65-year-old male is discussing an incidental CT finding with his primary care doctor in which it showed he has a 4.5cm AAA. He is concerned regarding the risk of rupture and has asked what the minimum size for surgery is if he remains asymptomatic and it does not grow more than 1cm per year.

a.   4cm.
b.   5cm.
c.   5.5cm.
d.   6cm.

19) A 67-year-old diabetic male attends his primary care doctor for a regular review. As part of the review, his feet are examined and he is noted to have several venous ulcers and a poorly healing wound on his left foot. Which of the following is not a risk factor for diabetic foot ulceration?

a. Altered foot shape.
b. Orthotic shoes.
c. Living alone.
d. Visual impairment.

20) Which of the following is not an early or intra-operative complication of vascular surgery?

a. Graft infection.
b. Reperfusion injury.
c. Trash foot.
d. Compartment syndrome.

21) Which of the following tests is not indicated in the investigation of leg ulcers?

a. Bloods tests including FBC, U&Es, clotting, glucose, ESR.
b. Duplex Doppler.
c. Microbiology swabs.
d. Tourniquet test.

22) A 56-year-old male is brought to the emergency department following a bookcase falling onto his right leg. The patient is in a large amount of pain despite opioid analgesia. There is pain on palpation of the limb and pain on passive stretching of the affected muscles. What is the most likely diagnosis?

a. Critical limb ischaemia.
b. Simple long bone fracture.
c. Femoral artery dissection.
d. Compartment syndrome.

23) A 65-year-old male attends his primary care doctor with a sudden loss of vision in his right eye, headache and a cramping pain in his jaw. On examination, he has scalp tenderness. He undergoes several tests which reveal a raised ESR and raised CRP. What is the most likely diagnosis?

a.   Thoracic outlet syndrome.

b.   Subclavian steal syndrome.

c.   Giant cell arteritis.

d.   Takayasu's arteritis.

Extended matching questions

Ankle Brachial Pressure Index

a. 0.

b. 0.15.

c. 0.35.

d. 0.6.

e. 0.8.

f. 1.0.

g. 1.4.

h. 2.0.

Match the most appropriate ABPI with each of the following patients.

1) A 72-year-old male presents to his primary care doctor with a 3-week history of pain in his left leg. He describes the pain as severe and he has used opioid analgesia with minimal effect. He is experiencing pain worst at night which is temporality relieved by hanging the leg out of bed. The pain occurs during the day even at rest. On examination, there is reduced sensation in the right foot but no gangrene is seen.

2) A 65-year-old diabetic presents to the clinic for vascular assessment following pain in his left leg. He undergoes ABPI measurements which the consultant believes reflects calcification of the artery.

3) A 45-year-old male attends the vascular clinic for mild pain in his right leg which is relieved by simple analgesia. The pain is sporadic and not linked to activity. The doctor reviewing the patient does not think this is a vascular issue and the ABPI is within the normal range.

4) A 66-year-old female smoker presents to her primary care doctor with pain on walking. She initially could walk 800m without pain but now experiences pain at 500m; however, this is relieved on rest and simple analgesia. The doctor believes she is experiencing mild intermittent claudication.

5) An 80-year-old male attends the vascular clinic with a 5-week history of a painful left leg. He experiences pain on walking short distances but does not experience rest pain. He is able to walk 150m before having to stop due to pain which is relieved by rest. On examination, there is no sign of gangrene or ulceration and an ABPI measurement shows moderate limb ischaemia with severe claudication.

Lower limb vascular pathology

a.   Chronic lower limb ischaemia.   e.   Lipodermatosclerosis.

b.   Critical limb ischaemia.   f.   Deep vein thrombosis (DVT).

c.   Leriche syndrome.   g.   Sciatica.

d.   Acute embolic ischaemia.   h.   Phlebitis.

Match the description with the most likely cause for their symptoms.

6)   A 68-year-old male presents to his primary care doctor with erectile dysfunction. He has also had cramping pain in his buttocks and thighs. On examination, femoral pulses are decreased bilaterally.

7)   A 66-year-old female attends her primary care doctor to enquire about an itchy brown pigmented area of skin on her leg; she is known to have varicose veins. On examination, varicosities are noted and a brown scaly region above her medial malleolus is seen.

8)   A 47-year-old female presents to the emergency department with a tender swollen left leg which started 24 hours ago; she has recently returned from a flight to Dubai. On examination, her left leg is 4cm larger than the right, there is tenderness along the deep venous system and left leg pitting oedema is noted.

9)   A 65-year-old presents to the vascular clinic with a 2-week history of pain in his right leg; the pain has been severe and he has used Oramorph® with little effect. He is experiencing the pain worst at night but is relieved when hanging his foot out of bed. Further questioning reveals he has had rest pain for the past 2 weeks. On examination, you note an area of wet gangrene on the medial malleolus.

10) A 67-year-old female with known AF presents to the emergency department with a painful, cold and pulseless right leg.

Vascular pathology

a.	Cervical rib.	e.	Filariasis.
b.	Buerger's disease.	f.	Klippel-Trenaunay syndrome.
c.	Subclavian steal syndrome.	g.	Stanford A aortic dissection.
d.	Renal artery stenosis.	h.	Stanford B aortic dissection.

Match the description of the patient with the most likely diagnosis.

11) A 19-year-old female presents to her primary care doctor with several episodes of her fingers changing colour in the cold weather. She explains that her fingers go initially white, then blue, and finally red before returning to their normal colour during cold weather. All other examination findings are normal.

12) A 65-year-old male attends his primary care doctor for a regular check-up. He is noted to have hypertension. The doctor is about to commence him on ramipril but remembers that this patient has a diagnosis which means ACE inhibitors are contraindicated.

13) A 69-year-old male presents to the emergency department with retrosternal chest pain which is of sudden onset and tearing in nature. The pain radiates to his arms. A CT of the chest shows the presence of an aortic dissection involving the aortic arch only.

14) A 26-year-old female presents to the vascular clinic following several episodes of collapse and a difference in blood pressure in each arm. An angiogram performed prior to her clinic visit shows retrograde vertebral artery flow on the right.

15) A 45-year-old female returns from travelling with bilateral swollen legs which started distally and is painless. The doctor assessing the patient suspects that she has secondary lymphoedema.

Investigations for vascular pathology

a.	Site auscultation.	e.	CTPA.
b.	Chest X-ray.	f.	MRI head.
c.	Ankle Brachial Pressure Index.	g.	Duplex ultrasound.
d.	CT abdomen.	h.	MSU.

Match the description of the patient with the most appropriate investigation.

16) A 56-year-old female presents with several tortuous veins on her right leg. They are not interfering with her daily life; however, she finds them unsightly and has an ache in her leg after long periods of standing. Her past medical history includes a previous DVT and hypertension.

17) A 78-year-old male presents to the emergency department with vague central abdominal pain radiating to the back. He has a history of hypercholesterolemia and hypertension.

18) A 26-year-old female presents to the emergency department with shortness of breath and mild chest pain following a recent diagnosis of a left leg DVT. ECG shows a sinus tachycardia.

19) A 78-year-old female presents to her primary care doctor with a deep wound to her leg which she says has been present for the past 2 weeks. On examination, you note a 3cm x 5cm ulcerated area which is well circumscribed and has a poorly healing base. Distal pulses are absent.

20) A 67-year-old male is seen in the vascular clinic following a recent TIA. He experienced a curtain falling across his eye which lasted for 5 minutes.

Complications of vascular surgery

a. Saphena varix.

b. Reperfusion injury.

c. Spinal cord ischaemia.

d. Acute mesenteric ischaemia.

e. Haemorrhage.

f. Endoleak.

g. Compartment syndrome.

h. Graft infection.

Match the description with the most likely complication that has occurred.

21) A 72-year-old male underwent a left femoral angioplasty for acute limb ischaemia. The nursing staff are concerned as he has noted some pain in his right leg which he is using Oramorph® to control and observations show he is tachycardic, tachypnoeic and hypotensive. You review the patient's bloods which show a new-onset acute renal failure which was not present 12 hours ago.

22) A 66-year-old male underwent an endovascular aneurysm repair 12 months ago. Prior to the surgery his aneurysm measured 6cm; however, on review it has now increased in size to 6.5cm.

23) A 56-year-old male is brought into resus following an explosion at a factory. The patient has multiple injuries including an arterial injury to his lower right leg. The patient is in a large amount of pain that does not fit with the clinical picture and pain on passive stretching of the affected muscles.

24) A 55-year-old male experiences weakness in both of his legs 48 hours after an abdominal aortic aneurysm repair. He reports no other symptoms and was fit and well prior to his operation.

25) A 68-year-old female presents to the vascular clinic for follow-up after a femoral distal bypass 2 years ago. She has recently noticed a large lump in her groin which is painful to touch and red. The area is not pulsatile and is warm to the touch.

Wells score for DVT

a. -1.   e. 4.
b. 1.   f. 5.
c. 2.   g. 6.
d. 3.   h. 7.

Calculate the Wells score for DVT on each of the following patients.

26) A 45-year-old female attends her primary care doctor with a swollen right leg which is hot and painful. She had a right hip replacement 3 weeks ago. On examination, her right leg is entirely swollen, pitting oedema is present in the right leg only and her right calf measures 8cm compared with 4cm on the left.

27) A 56-year-old male with a previous DVT presents to the emergency department with a swollen right leg. On examination, you note the right leg is swollen, there is localised tenderness along the deep venous system and collateral non-varicose superficial veins are present. The right calf is 2cm larger than the left.

28) A 26-year-old female attends the emergency department with a right leg swelling. She noted this started 2 days ago. She is concerned about DVT as her father has had a recent diagnosis following his cancer treatment. On examination, a 5cm erythematous patch is noted on her left calf which is hot and tender. She has a temperature of 38.2°C. The right calf is 2cm bigger than the left and the whole right leg is swollen.

29) A 29-year-old male presents to the emergency department with a swollen left leg. He is currently receiving treatment for lymphoma. On examination, the left calf is 6cm larger than the right and the left leg is entirely swollen. There is tenderness along the deep venous system and pitting oedema on the left only.

30) A 20-year-old female presents to the emergency department with a swollen right limb. She recently fractured her right leg and has been immobilised since this time. The right calf is 4cm larger than the left and the entire limb is swollen. The doctor believes this patient has a DVT.

Management of acute lower limb ischaemia

a.	Amputation.	e.	Embolectomy.
b.	Best medical therapy.	f.	No treatment.
c.	Palliative care.	g.	Bypass.
d.	Fasciotomy.	h.	Anticoagulation.

Match the most appropriate treatment for each patient.

31) A 65-year-old female presents to the emergency department with a severely painful left limb for the past 3 hours. She has a past medical history of peripheral vascular disease. She has not been able to move her leg for the past 2 hours. On examination, she has an absent capillary refill, paralysis and loss of sensation in the left leg. Pulses are not palpable and Doppler scans are unable to obtain a signal. The limb has signs of fixed mottling and tense swollen fascial compartments.

32) A 65-year-old male with known AF presents to the emergency department with a painful, cold and pulseless left leg.

33) A 75-year-old male smoker attends his primary care doctor with a cramping pain in his left leg after walking. The pain starts after walking 500m. He previously could walk 800m before he had this pain 12 months ago. The pain resolves at rest and with simple analgesia.

34) A 76-year-old male attends the vascular clinic with symptoms of moderate limb ischaemia. An angiogram has shown multilevel disease and a long occlusion of the superficial femoral artery.

35) A 65-year-old male is brought to the emergency department following trauma to his left leg. The patient is in pain despite opioid analgesia; there is pain on limb palpation and pain on passive stretching.

Types of ulceration

a. Arterial ulcer.
b. Venous ulcer.
c. Neuropathic ulcer.
d. Aphthous ulcer.

e. Cushing's ulcer.
f. Curling's ulcer.
g. Marjolin ulcer.
h. Callous ulcer.

Match the description of the patient with the most likely diagnosis.

36) A 65-year-old male presents to his primary care doctor with a large ulcer over his medial malleolus. On examination, the ulcer measures 5cm x 8cm and has a shallow base with sloping edges and granulation tissue is present.

37) A 67-year-old female presents to her primary care doctor with ulceration on her left foot. The wound appears to be deep and is located on the dorsum of the toes. It is deep with well-defined edges and has a cuff of callous. The foot is otherwise normal and bounding pulses are felt. The ABPI is normal.

38) A 68-year-old male presents to the vascular clinic following a 2-week history of a poorly healing wound on the dorsum of his left foot. The wound is deep with a well-demarcated border. The base appears to be necrotic. Distal pulses are absent and his foot feels cool to the touch.

39) A 71-year-old female presents to her primary care doctor as she is concerned about the changing nature of one of her venous ulcers. The ulcer has been increasing steadily in size and bleeds easily on contact. She has noted increased pain. On examination, the ulcer appears flat with hardened and elevated edges.

40) A 56-year-old male is brought into resus with severe burns to his face, chest and arms. He is transferred to the burns unit for further treatment. What type of ulcer is a complication of this type of injury?

Management of abdominal aortic aneurysms (AAAs)

a.   Ultrasound in 6 months.   e.   Urgent elective repair.

b.   Ultrasound in 12 months.   f.   Emergency repair.

c.   Ultrasound in 18 months.   g.   Elective open repair.

d.   Ultrasound in 24 months.   h.   Elective EVAR procedure.

Match the most appropriate follow-up for each of the following patients.

41)   A 68-year-old male attends for routine AAA screening and is found to have a 4.8cm aneurysm. He does not have any symptoms.

42)   A 72-year-old male enters the emergency department hypotensive, tachycardic and pale. He has had a vague central abdominal pain radiating to his back for 12 hours. He is stabilised in resus and a CT scans shows a ruptured aortic aneurysm.

43)   A 70-year-old male attends the vascular clinic for routine follow-up for his AAA. His most recent scan shows the aneurysm has increased by 1.5cm in 12 months.

44)   A 70-year-old male is found to have a 5.5cm infra-renal AAA. It is located 4cm below the renal arteries.

45)   A 66-year-old male attends for AAA screening and is found to have a 3.2cm aneurysm. He has no other symptoms.

Short answer questions

1) A 75-year-old male presents to the vascular clinic with a 3-week history of pain in his left leg. The pain has been severe and he has tried opioid analgesia with little effect. The pain is worst at night but is relieved when hanging his foot out of bed. On examination, his left leg is cold to the touch, capillary refill is reduced and skin damage is evident over pressure areas.

a. What is the underlying diagnosis?   1 mark
b. State two differences between this diagnosis and intermittent   2 marks
    claudication.
c. Name four risk factors for developing this condition.   2 marks
d. Name two investigations that may be requested.   2 marks
e. Specify three treatment options for this patient.   3 marks

2) A 65-year-old male is seen by his primary care doctor following an ultrasound scan as part of the Abdominal Aortic Aneurysm Screening Programme. He is found to have a 3.5cm aneurysm and the primary care doctor would like to discuss the options for future management.

a. Name four causes of an AAA.   2 marks
b. Describe two ways that aneurysms can be classified.   2 marks
c. Specify four indications for surgical intervention for an AAA.   2 marks
d. What is the UK Abdominal Aortic Aneurysm Screening Programme   2 marks
    and which patients will receive further follow-up?
e. Name two sites other than the aorta that aneurysms can be   2 marks
    commonly found.

3) A 32-year-old female attends her primary care doctor surgery with a swollen right leg. She is currently receiving treatment for breast cancer. On examination, the right calf is entirely swollen and 7cm larger than the left. There is tenderness along the deep venous system and pitting oedema on the right only.

a. Name two signs and two symptoms the patient may experience. 2 marks

b. Specify the three broad areas of Virchow's triad and provide one 3 marks example of each category.

c. What is the patient's Wells score? 1 mark

d. State one treatment option for this patient. 1 mark

e. Describe three complications this patient may develop. 3 marks

4) A 65-year-old female presents to her primary care doctor with a wound over her medial malleolus. It has been present for the past 2 weeks. On examination, the wound measures 5cm x 8cm and has a shallow base with sloping edges and granulation tissue is present. She is diagnosed as having a venous ulcer.

a. Name the three common lower limb ulcers. 3 marks

b. Specify two investigations for this patient. 2 marks

c. Describe three chronic venous changes that may be evident on 3 marks examination.

d. State one treatment option for this patient. 1 mark

e. After 4 months of treatment, the community nurse notes that the 1 mark ulcer appears to have developed raised, rolled edges with a large amount of granulation tissue. What condition is the nurse concerned about?

5) A 72-year-old male with AF presents to the emergency department with a painful, cold and pulseless left leg.

a. Name four causes of acute limb ischaemia.   2 marks

b. Specify the six classical signs of acute limb ischaemia.   3 marks

c. Name two investigations that could be requested in this patient.   1 mark

d. State one definitive treatment that could be offered.   1 mark

e. Describe the three subgroups of limb viability for the acute ischaemic limb.   3 marks

6) A 69-year-old male presents to the emergency department with symptoms suggestive of an aortic dissection. His symptoms and examination findings are subsequently confirmed on imaging.

a. Specify two symptoms and two signs this patient may describe.   4 marks

b. What is the aetiology of this condition?   1 mark

c. Describe the two classification systems of this condition.   2 marks

d. State two investigations that could be requested in this patient.   2 marks

e. What is the management option for a patient with a descending aorta dissection which does not involve the aortic arch?   1 mark

7) A 20-year-old male is taken to the emergency department following a stabbing in his right groin by a local gang. He has a profusely bleeding wound which you believe is arterial in nature.

a. Name two immediate actions that are needed for this patient.   2 marks

b. What three structures may be damaged from this injury?   3 marks

c. Name two signs that may lead you to suspect a vascular injury.   2 marks

d. Specify one method of surgically treating this vascular injury.   1 mark

e. Name two complications the patient may experience as a result of a vascular injury.   2 marks

8) A 75-year-old male presents to the emergency department with severe central abdominal pain radiating to the lower back which suddenly started 2 hours ago. On examination, he is pale, hypotensive and tachycardic, with a prolonged capillary refill time at 6 seconds and the absence of a left femoral pulse.

a. What is the underlying diagnosis? — 1 mark

b. Name six immediate management actions for this patient. — 3 marks

c. What is permissive hypotension and how may this be beneficial for this patient? — 2 marks

d. How can this condition be surgically treated? — 2 marks

e. Name two complications following the procedure. — 2 marks

9) A 30-year-old female asks her primary care doctor to review several prominent veins on her right calf. On examination, she has multiple varicosities on the right leg and a positive tourniquet test. She has recently given birth. The doctor diagnoses her with varicose veins.

a. Describe the classification of varicose veins. — 2 marks

b. Name two risk factors for developing varicose. — 2 marks

c. Specify two common sites for varicosities to occur. — 2 marks

d. Name three treatments that can be offered to this patient. — 3 marks

e. If this patient was planning to have further children, what would you recommend regarding her treatment? — 1 mark

10) A 60-year-old male is referred to the vascular clinic for likely carotid artery disease following a recent hospital admission.

a.	Name four common presentations of carotid artery disease.	4 marks
b.	What is the underlying pathology of carotid disease?	2 marks
c.	Name one initial investigation that is indicated to assess the carotid arteries.	1 mark
d.	If the above investigation showed a stenosis of 85%, what would be the most appropriate treatment option?	1 mark
e.	Name four medical therapies that can be used in this patient.	2 marks

11) A 62-year-old diabetic female presents to her primary care doctor for a routine review. On examination, she has ulceration on her left medial malleolus with surrounding cellulitis. The doctor is concerned as the ulceration was not present 12 weeks ago. She has a loss of pinprick sensation and an absent dorsalis pedis.

a.	Name four aetiological factors for the development of a diabetic foot condition.	4 marks
b.	Specify four risk factors for diabetic foot ulceration.	2 marks
c.	State four general measures to reduce the risk of developing diabetic foot ulceration.	2 marks
d.	State two medical measures to reduce the risk of developing diabetic foot ulceration.	1 mark
e.	Explain why the ABPI may be falsely elevated in diabetic patients.	1 mark

12) A 40-year-old male is brought into the emergency department following a crush injury by a bookcase. The patient has multiple injuries including an open tibial fracture to his right leg. The patient is in severe pain that does not correlate with the clinical picture and pain on passive stretching of the affected muscles.

a. What is the underlying diagnosis?   1 mark
b. Name four causes of this condition.   2 marks
c. Specify three early and three late signs of this condition.   3 marks
d. If suspected, what two treatment options should be performed?   2 marks
e. Name two sequelae of a lower limb compartment syndrome.   2 marks

13) A 50-year-old male returns from travelling in India with a right swollen leg which started distally and is painless. He has a mild fever and inguinal lymphadenopathy. The doctor assessing the patient suspects that he has secondary lymphoedema.

a. State the difference between primary and secondary lymphoedema. 2 marks
b. Name two causes of primary and two causes of secondary   2 marks
    lymphoedema.
c. Give two differential diagnoses of lymphoedema.   2 marks
d. Give two investigations that are used if the diagnosis is in doubt or 2 marks
    prior to lymphatic reconstruction surgery.
e. Give two management options for lymphoedema.   2 marks

Chapter 4

Breast surgery
QUESTIONS

Single best answer questions

1) BRCA 1 and BRCA 2 have not been linked to which cancer?

a. Breast.
b. Ovarian.
c. Pancreatic.
d. Gastric.

2) At what age does the national screening program for breast cancer begin?

a. 55.
b. 65.
c. 50.
d. 45.

3) A 30-year-old female presents with right-sided breast pain of 3 weeks' duration. On examination, she is tender on palpation of the chest and there is some chest swelling. What is the most likely diagnosis?

a. Costochondritis.
b. Tietze syndrome.
c. Breast cancer.
d. Lipoma.

4) An elderly female presents with a scaly erythematous rash over her left nipple. What is the most likely diagnosis?

a. Breast cyst.
b. Paget's disease.
c. Fat necrosis.
d. Eczema.

5) The majority of breast lymph drains to which area?

a. Axillary nodes.
b. Parasternal nodes.
c. Opposite breast.
d. Sub-diaphragmatic nodes.

6) An 11-year-old male presents to the breast clinic with gynaecomastia. What is the most likely cause?

a. Breast cancer.
b. Prolactinoma.
c. Iatrogenic.
d. Physiological.

7) Which hormone stimulates milk production in the breast?

a. Luteinising hormone.
b. Oxytocin.
c. Follicle-stimulating hormone.
d. Prolactin.

8) What marks the lateral border of the breast?

a. Mid-axillary line.
b. Anterior axillary line.
c. Posterior axillary line.
d. 6th rib.

9) The mammary gland is attached to skin by which of the following?

a. Internal intercostals.
b. External intercostals.
c. Suspensory ligaments of Cooper.
d. Pectoralis major.

10) Which of the following arteries does not contribute to the blood supply of the breast?

a. Internal thoracic.
b. Posterior intercostal.
c. Thyrocervical.
d. Lateral thoracic.

11) Before milk is produced in preparation for breastfeeding, what substance is first secreted?

a. Mucus.
b. Colostrum.
c. Blood.
d. Plasma.

12) Which of the following is not classically a sign of breast cancer?

a. Thickened skin.
b. Nipple inversion.
c. Nipple deviation.
d. Breast pain.

13) Which hormone stimulates milk ejection from the breast?

a. Prolactin.
b. Oxytocin.
c. Luteinising hormone.
d. Follicle-stimulating hormone.

14) What is the inferior border of the breast?

a. 6th rib.
b. Subcostal plane.
c. Xiphoid process.
d. 7th rib.

15) What relation does pectoralis major have to the breast?

a. Deep.
b. Superficial.
c. Lateral.
d. None of the above.

16) Where does the majority of breast venous blood drain to?

a. Axillary vein.
b. Basilic vein.
c. Accessory hemiazygos.
d. Oesophageal plexus.

17) The nipple classically lies on which dermatome?

a. C3.
b. L2.
c. T10.
d. T4.

18) The thoracic duct drains into which of the following?

a. Right subclavian vein.
b. Superior vena cava.
c. Left subclavian vein.
d. Left brachiocephalic vein.

19) Which of the following is not a cause of gynaecomastia?

a. Testicular cancer.
b. Klinefelter syndrome.
c. Adrenal cancer.
d. Bowel cancer.

20) In the UK, what percentage of breast cancers occurs in men?

a. <1%.
b. 1-10%.
c. 10-20%.
d. 20-25%.

21) Which imaging technique exposes patients to radiation?

a. Ultrasound scan.
b. MRI scan.
c. Mammogram.
d. None of the above.

22) First-line treatment options for cyclical breast pain do not include which of the following?

a. Better fitting day bra.
b. Combined oral contraceptive pill.
c. Ibuprofen.
d. Night support bra.

23) A 35-year-old (pre-menopausal) female is to be started on hormonal therapy for breast cancer. Which agent is the most appropriate?

a.   Anastrozole.
b.   Tamoxifen.
c.   Exemestane.
d.   Letrozole.

Extended matching questions

Breast pathology

a. Traumatic necrosis.

b. Breast cancer.

c. Mastitis.

d. Skin cancer.

e. Lipoma.

f. Breast abscess.

g. Fibroadenoma.

h. Breast cyst.

Match the description of the patient with the most likely diagnosis.

1) A 32-year-old breastfeeding mother presents with a 2-day history of a painful right breast. On examination, there is a wedge-shaped area of redness and swelling, which is very tender. She is also tachycardic.

2) A 24-year-old presents with a small 5mm left-sided breast lump. It is soft, non-tender and superficial.

3) A 36-year-old mother presents to her primary care doctor for the second time with a swollen left breast. She had been given antibiotics for this 1 week ago, which has helped with her pain and fever; however, the breast is still swollen and now feels firm.

4) A 52-year-old peri-menopausal female presents to her primary care doctor with a painful lump in her right breast. On examination, it is large and round. She had a similar lump like this previously.

5) An 80-year-old lady presents with an itchy left nipple; there is a red, dry patch surrounding the nipple.

Breast investigations

a.   Biopsy.
b.   CT scan.
c.   Mammogram.
d.   Bone scan.

e.   Ductogram.
f.   Ultrasound scan.
g.   Genetic testing.
h.   Abdominal ultrasound.

Select the initial most appropriate investigation.

6)   A 70-year-old female presents to the clinic having felt a mass in her left breast. Her mammogram shows no abnormality. Her USS shows a 3cm lesion in the upper outer quadrant.

7)   A 59-year-old female is called for screening by her local hospital.

8)   A 27-year-old female presents with a right-sided mobile breast mass.

9)   An 82-year-old female presents to the emergency department with confusion and headaches. On examination, she has a large left-sided breast mass.

10) A 64-year-old female with a recent diagnosis of breast cancer presents with chest pain. She has a heart rate of 110 beats per minute, blood pressure 120/90mmHg, respiratory rate 20 and a saturation of 88% on air. Her chest X-ray is normal.

Brachial plexus

a. Axillary nerve.
b. Long thoracic nerve.
c. Median nerve.
d. Ulnar nerve.

e. Thoracodorsal nerve.
f. Subscapular nerve.
g. Radial nerve.
h. Intercostobrachial nerve.

What is the most likely structure that has been injured?

11) A 66-year-old female who underwent axillary node clearance for breast cancer returns to the clinic having noticed a numb patch whilst shaving her underarm.

12) You examine a 75-year-old female who had a mastectomy 25 years ago. You notice she finds it difficult to extend and adduct her arm.

13) A 17-year-old male presents with shoulder pain and deformity after a rugby tackle. He does not have any sensation over the deltoid area when you examine him.

14) An elderly male presents after a fall with a swollen and painful right arm. His X-ray shows a fracture in the mid shaft of the humerus.

15) A 70-year-old female presents with a rash on her back. Whilst examining her, you notice that her scapulae are asymmetrical. She tells you she had some "glands removed years ago" and she has been like this ever since.

Targeted treatments

a.   Oestrogen receptor.
b.   Progesterone receptor.
c.   Herceptin®.
d.   Tamoxifen.

e.   Aromatase inhibitors.
f.   Radiotherapy.
g.   Testosterone receptor.
h.   Methotrexate.

Match the description with the most likely answer.

16) A 35-year-old female is taking a tablet for therapy of her breast cancer. This therapy antagonises oestrogen in the breast but can cause endometrial hyperplasia.

17) You see a 70-year-old female in the clinic for regular follow-up. She has advanced breast cancer and is on hormone therapy for oestrogen receptor-positive breast cancer. What is she most likely taking?

18) Trastuzumab is more commonly known by which name?

19) Triple-negative breast cancers do not express oestrogen receptors, Herceptin genes and which other receptor?

20) You receive a report of a breast cancer that over expresses human epidermal growth factor receptor 2. Which treatment would you consider?

Breast complaints

a.   Routine breast referral.
b.   Urgent breast referral.
c.   Referral to dermatology.
d.   Reassurance alone.
e.   Analgesia alone.
f.   Primary care doctor follow-up.
g.   Urgent referral to the emergency department.
h.   Physiotherapy referral.

Select the correct next step in management.

21)   A 75-year-old female presents to her primary care doctor with right nipple discharge. She is usually fit and well.

22)   A 25-year-old female presents to her primary care doctor with concerns regarding breast cancer. She has not noticed any lumps; however, both her mother and grandmother have had breast cancer.

23)   A 20-year-old female presents to her primary care doctor with painful breasts. She has noticed that this happens approximately once a month. When this occurs her breasts feel "lumpier" and tender. Your examination is normal.

24)   A 30-year-old breastfeeding mother presents with breast pain. On examination, the breast is swollen and red. She looks pale and unwell. You take her observations and her temperature is 39°C, her BP is 75/50mmHg and heart rate is 110 bpm.

25)   A 45-year-old male presents to you after noticing his right breast looks different than his left. On examination, you feel a small round lump that is fixed and the skin is puckered.

Family history

a.   Routine breast referral.
b.   Urgent breast referral.
c.   Referral to dermatology.
d.   Reassurance alone.

e.   Analgesia alone.
f.   Primary care doctor follow-up.
g.   Urgent referral to the
     emergency department.
h.   Physiotherapy referral.

What would be the next step in management?

26)   A 34-year-old female presents to you having felt something whilst shaving her right underarm. On examination, you feel two small lumps when palpating against the chest wall.

27)   A 25-year-old female presents to her primary care doctor with a new right-sided breast lump. On examination, it feels soft, round and non-tender.

28)   A 35-year-old male presents to his primary care doctor with concerns regarding cancer. His father was diagnosed with breast cancer at age 55, but no other family members that he is aware of.

29)   A 39-year-old female presents to you after news her mother has been diagnosed with breast cancer at age 75. Her mother is otherwise fit and well and no-one else in the family has had breast cancer. She would like to know if she needs any "special tests" to ensure she does not have a "bad gene".

30)   A female presents to her primary care doctor dissatisfied. She was previously reassured that she does not need further investigations after her mum was diagnosed with breast cancer at the age of 42. She says she has been thinking about it a lot recently and would like a second opinion.

Benign breast conditions

a.	Thrombophlebitis.	e.	Periductal mastitis.
b.	Fat necrosis.	f.	Gynaecomastia.
c.	Duct ectasia.	g.	Intraductal papilloma.
d.	Intertrigo.	h.	Breast cyst.

Match the description of the patient with the most likely diagnosis.

31) A 45-year-old female presents to you with left-sided nipple discharge. She says it is sometimes bloodstained and can be sore. On examination, you note a 1cm lump beneath the areola. The patient otherwise feels well and observations are normal.

32) A 45-year-old female comes to see you a month after a road traffic accident where she was the driver. Since then she has developed a lump over her right upper breast. When you examine it, this feels firm and seems to be made up of multiple small lumps.

33) A 50-year-old female attends the clinic as she has noticed some nipple discharge. The discharge colour and consistency can vary, from clear to thick and creamy. She denies any pain.

34) You see an overweight 65-year-old female on a home visit complaining of pain under her breasts. She lives alone with once a day carers. When you examine her breasts, you notice sore, wet, red areas on the underside of both breasts. You ask her how long this has been there but she does not know, as she struggles to wash and self-care.

35) You see a female who has had a recent biopsy in the breast clinic. Since then she has been experiencing pain when putting her bra on and has noticed some redness and swelling of the breast. On examination, she has a streak of redness and swelling, and on palpation it has a cord-like feel.

Treatment complications

a.	Thrombophlebitis.	e.	Cellulitis.
b.	Allergic/anaphylactic reaction.	f.	Abscess.
c.	Haematoma.	g.	Seroma.
d.	Eczema.	h.	Intertrigo.

Match the description of the patient with the most likely diagnosis.

36) A 45-year-old female has had a wide local excision for a breast cancer. You are the on-call doctor and you have been called to see her due to increasing pain around her wound site. Her observations show mild tachycardia. You remove the dressing to find the wound is red, swollen and tender.

37) A 19-year-old female with a history of depression and asthma has just returned from theatre. She has been complaining of pain so the nurse has given the analgesia prescribed. She has had removal of a large fibroadenoma. She alerts the nursing staff as she has started vomiting and feels unwell. Soon after she opens her bowels and has diarrhoea.

38) A female has returned to you in clinic 1 week after a mastectomy and axillary node clearance. She has noticed a swelling in the same breast that seems to be slowly increasing in size. It was initially non-tender but is now getting uncomfortable when rubbing against her underarm. When you examine her breast it feels soft and fluctuant.

39) A 35-year-old female presents 3 days after a breast biopsy. Since then she has developed a red rash around the whole breast. It is sore and itchy and today started weeping.

40) A 55-year-old female attends the day unit to begin chemotherapy. She has a cannula inserted and has the process explained to her. The infusion begins but 5 minutes in she calls the nurse, as she is feeling very hot. She suddenly becomes very short of breath and collapses.

Clinic findings

a.	Fibroadenoma.	e.	Duct ectasia.
b.	Phyllodes tumour.	f.	Pituitary adenoma.
c.	Lobular carcinoma.	g.	Ductal carcinoma *in situ*.
d.	Prolactinoma.	h.	Metastatic disease.

Match the description of the patient with the most likely diagnosis.

41) A female presents to you with one-sided white nipple discharge. On examination, you find she is hursuit and has bad acne.

42) A 52-year-old menopausal female comes to you complaining of nipple discharge. On examination, the nipple is retracted. She is a lifelong smoker but is otherwise fit and well.

43) A histology report has come back for a patient you saw in a 2-week wait clinic. This patient presented with a firm mass which had increased in size very rapidly and caused severe deformity of the breast. You were awaiting histology to see if this was a benign or malignant growth.

44) Histology returns for a 50-year-old patient you have seen in the clinic. She attended routine screening mammography where calcifications were seen. She was invited for biopsy and further assessment. Histology shows that there is no invasion of the ductal basement membrane.

45) A 62-year-old female presents to your clinic via her primary care doctor. She has had an ongoing skin rash over her right breast for 6 weeks that is not improving. The doctor has prescribed a course of flucloxacillin and various topical creams; however, this has not improved her symptoms. The skin is now more irritable and painful and the rash has spread to the left breast. She has had previous surgery for breast cancer removal 5 years ago.

Short answer questions

1) A 64-year-old female presents with severe upper back pain. She has a history of hypertension, AF and metastatic breast cancer. She is currently taking warfarin. When the ambulance arrived they noted that she had been faecally incontinent. You are concerned about spinal cord compression. On examination, you find the patient has upper motor neurone signs in her legs.

a. Which two other cancers commonly metastasise to the spine? 2 marks
b. Name four upper motor neurone signs in the lower limbs. 4 marks
c. Other than analgesia, name one treatment to be given as soon as possible. 1 mark
d. What image modality would you urgently request? 1 mark
e. Once diagnosed, state two further treatment options. 2 marks

2) After undergoing surgery for removal of a breast cancer, a 55-year-old female has radiotherapy to her axilla. She subsequently develops a swollen arm on the same side and comes to see you in clinic.

a. Which medium is radiotherapy delivered in? 1 mark
b. List six acute side effects of radiotherapy. 3 marks
c. List six long-term side effects of radiotherapy. 3 marks
d. What is the most likely cause of this patient's arm swelling? 1 mark
e. What test should be carried out before you make your suspected diagnosis and what are you looking for? 2 marks

3) A 55-year-old female undergoing breast cancer treatment presents to hospital with her husband. He says that over the past 2 days she has been more confused. Today she has been vomiting and holding her stomach. You think she may have an electrolyte imbalance.

a. What is the most likely imbalance she has? 1 mark
b. State four other electrolyte imbalances for prolonged vomiting. 4 marks
c. What is the first step in treatment? 1 mark
d. Other than basic observations, what other monitoring device may be 2 marks
   useful in this situation and why?
e. What medication could be administered once fluid resuscitation has 2 marks
   been established and how does it work?

4) A 74-year-old female is admitted with increased shortness of breath, a productive cough and generalised weakness. She has a history of AF and advanced breast cancer and is currently having palliative chemotherapy. You see her in the emergency department and take her observations: blood pressure 110/70mmHg, respiratory rate 25 breaths per minute, pulse 110 beats per minute, oxygen saturation 88%, and temperature 38.4°C. You suspect a diagnosis of sepsis.

a. What six investigations would be useful in this patient? 3 marks
b. What six steps would you use to manage her sepsis? 3 marks
c. What else are you concerned about given the history? 1 mark
d. Blood tests show a WCC of 2.0 x 10^9/L, Hb 74g/L, platelets 50 x 10^9/L 1 mark
   and neutrophils 0.6 x 10^9/L. Which team would you call for advice?
e. She has now received full management for her sepsis but still remains 2 marks
   unwell and has been deemed appropriate for ward-based care only.
   Her family are not with her and cannot be contacted. Your senior
   colleague discusses the indications for DNACPR forms with you and
   begins to fill one out. Can this be done without the family's consent?

5) A 52-year-old female who has been recently diagnosed with breast cancer comes to the emergency department with her husband with a difficulty in breathing. She says that it has been getting worse over the past 2 weeks and she feels very tired. Her observations show a respiratory rate of 20 with normal saturations, temperature and pulse. She has no other medical problems. You listen to her chest and find that you struggle to hear breath sounds over the left lower zone. On percussion this area is dull.

a. What do you suspect? 2 marks

b. Which investigation may confirm your diagnosis in the emergency 2 marks
department?

c. What would you expect to see? 2 marks

d. As this patient is symptomatic, what procedure would you consider 2 marks
for relieving symptoms and confirming the diagnosis?

e. On sample analysis, state two things you expect to find. 2 marks

6) A female who is taking tamoxifen for oestrogen receptor-positive breast cancer presents to the emergency department with a painful leg. She says her lower leg has been very painful over the past 24 hours and is now starting to swell. On examination, she is tender and has pitting oedema. You measure a 4cm difference between the two calves.

a. What diagnosis do you suspect? 1 mark

b. Name five other differential diagnoses. 5 marks

c. What would you use to assess for your first diagnosis? 1 mark

d. State the most appropriate imaging to confirm the diagnosis. 1 mark

e. Specify two initial treatment options. 2 marks

7) A 72-year-old patient with known advanced breast cancer presents to the emergency department unable to weight bear. She reports that she was standing in the kitchen preparing dinner when she suddenly fell to the floor. She complains of pain in the left upper thigh when she tries to move her leg. On examination, she is unable to move her left leg due to pain and her left leg looks different to her right. Sensation and pulses are intact.

a. What do you suspect may have occurred? 1 mark
b. What three things may you find on examination? 3 marks
c. What is the underlying process responsible for this event? 2 marks
d. Which specialty should this be referred to? 1 mark
e. What three other treatments should be considered in patients with this pathology? 3 marks

8) A patient with advanced metastatic cancer presents to you with shortness of breath and chest pain. This has increased over the past few weeks and is worse on bending over. You carry out a chest X-ray and it shows a large right-sided mass, which appears bigger than his previous chest X-ray 2 months ago.

a. What is the most likely cause? 1 mark
b. Name four other signs you would look for. 4 marks
c. What could you ask the patient to do to help your examination of these signs? 1 mark
d. How would you structure the management of this patient? 1 mark
e. State three treatment options for this pathology. 3 marks

9) A patient with known breast cancer presents with a painful, swollen arm. This has developed over the past 2 days but she is now feeling more short of breath. She has no infective symptoms and examination of the chest is normal. You suspect upper limb DVT that may have caused a PE.

a. What is your first choice of treatment?   1 mark
b. Should this be given before or after confirming the diagnosis with   2 marks
    imaging and explain your decision?
c. How does this treatment work?   3 marks
d. Does this treatment require blood level monitoring?   2 marks
e. When prescribing venous thromboembolism prophylaxis for ward-   2 marks
    based patients, state two other measures that must be considered
    other than renal function.

10) A 65-year-old female presents to the primary care doctor with fatigue and loss of appetite. She has had previous treatment for breast cancer and her follow-up scan 2 weeks ago shows no recurrence. You decide to do some blood tests to search for a medical cause.

a. What six blood tests would you consider?   3 marks
b. These tests all come back within normal limits. You ask her more   1 mark
    about her tiredness and she says she has been having trouble
    sleeping recently. She finds herself taking a long time to get to sleep
    but waking daily at 4am. What diagnosis should you consider?
c. Name two diagnostic tools that could be useful.   2 marks
d. If after conservative measures you decided this patient needs medical   2 marks
    treatment, what would be your first choice in class of medication and
    provide one example?
e. What two questions must you remember to ask?   2 marks

11) You see a patient in clinic 1 week after a mastectomy. She complains of some pain around the area of the scar. On examination, the wound is intact; however, there is some erythema and it is warm and tender to touch. You suspect cellulitis. The patient has no allergies.

a.	What is the most likely organism causing this reaction?	2 marks
b.	What would be an appropriate first-line antibiotic?	2 marks
c.	If the patient thought she was allergic to penicillin but could not recall the reaction, would you prescribe her a penicillin?	2 marks
d.	What alternative antibiotic class could be used if this patient was allergic to penicillin?	2 marks
e.	You receive a call from the emergency department 3 days later to inform you she has presented to the department septic. The wound has broken down and is exuding pus. What two microbiological investigations would be appropriate?	2 marks

12) A 60-year-old female is referred to the breast clinic by her primary care doctor after feeling a breast lump. You examine her and feel a mass in the upper outer quadrant of the right breast. No lymphadenopathy is felt.

a.	Name six factors that increase a person's risk of breast cancer.	3 marks
b.	Name four examination findings of a breast lump that would suggest malignancy.	2 marks
c.	State the four areas breast cancer is most likely to metastasise.	2 marks
d.	Which two genetic markers increase the risk for breast cancer?	2 marks
e.	What imaging would be appropriate for an initial assessment?	1 mark

13) A 43-year-old female presents to her primary care doctor with a breast lump. She has noticed some blood-stained nipple discharge over the past 2 days. She feels well in herself; her only other health problem is hypertension. You examine her and find a small, non-tender 5mm lump behind her right areola. You suspect an intraductal papilloma.

a. Where should you now refer this patient?   1 mark

b. What will the patient receive once referred?   1 mark

c. Name two types of biopsy techniques that may be used.   2 marks

d. State three lifestyle factors that can affect wound healing.   3 marks

e. Name three medical conditions that can affect wound healing.   3 marks

Chapter 5

Urology
QUESTIONS

Single best answer questions

1) What is the commonest type of testicular tumour found in younger men (aged 20-30 years)?

a. Non-seminomatous germ-cell tumours.
b. Lymphoma.
c. Seminoma.
d. Sarcoma.

2) The main feature of which condition is an abnormally sustained erection unrelated to sexual stimulation?

a. Peyronie's disease.
b. Phimosis.
c. Priapism.
d. Paraphimosis.

3) What is the most common type of renal stone?

a. Uric acid.
b. Cystine.
c. Calcium phosphate.
d. Calcium oxalate.

4) What is the usual treatment for an uncomplicated UTI in males?

a. 3 days of oral antibiotics.
b. 7 days of oral antibiotics.
c. 10 days of oral antibiotics.
d. Analgesia and reassurance.

5) Which type of renal tumour is most common in childhood?

a. Renal cell carcinoma.
b. Transitional cell carcinoma of the renal pelvis.
c. Nephroblastoma.
d. Clear cell tumour.

6) What is the most appropriate initial medication for lower urinary tract symptoms due to benign prostatic enlargement?

a. Alpha-receptor antagonist, e.g. tamsulosin.
b. Beta-receptor antagonist, e.g. bisoprolol.
c. 5-alpha-reductase inhibitor, e.g. finasteride.
d. Antimuscarinic, e.g. solifenacin.

7) Which muscle contributes most to the ejection of urine from the bladder?

a. Cremaster.
b. Detrusor.
c. Puborectalis.
d. Iliococcygeus.

8) Which infective illness is most associated with epididymo-orchitis?

a. Influenza.
b. Meningitis.
c. Mumps.
d. Croup.

9) What is the most likely cause for painless haematuria in the United Kingdom?

a. Ureteric colic.
b. Squamous cell carcinoma of the bladder.
c. Transitional cell carcinoma of the urethra.
d. Transitional cell carcinoma of the bladder.

10) What is the most common organic cause for erectile dysfunction?

a. Diabetes mellitus.
b. Right-sided heart failure.
c. Prostate cancer.
d. Psychological.

11) Which condition is characterised by penile plaques causing curvature of the erect penis?

a.   Nesbitt's disorder.
b.   Fournier's gangrene.
c.   Hydatid of Morgagni.
d.   Peyronie's disease.

12) Since the birth of her child by vaginal delivery a female reports leakage of urine during exercise, coughing or laughing. What is the likeliest diagnosis?

a.   Overactive bladder.
b.   Stress urinary incontinence.
c.   Prolapsed uterus.
d.   Vesico-vaginal fistula.

13) How should painless haematuria be managed in the first instance?

a.   Flexible cystoscopy and renal tract ultrasound.
b.   CT KUB.
c.   Flexible cystoscopy and bladder biopsies.
d.   Rigid cystoscopy and diathermy to tumours.

14) Which of the following is not a recognised cause for a raised PSA?

a.   Prostate adenocarcinoma.
b.   Benign prostatic enlargement.
c.   Urinary tract infection.
d.   Excessive cheese consumption.

15) Which type of tumour is typically found with penile cancers?

a. Transitional cell carcinoma.
b. Squamous cell carcinoma.
c. Adenocarcinoma.
d. Lymphoma.

16) What is the treatment usually offered to men with locally advanced prostate cancer without metastasis?

a. Hormonal therapy.
b. Radiotherapy.
c. Radical prostatectomy.
d. PSA surveillance.

17) A middle-aged female reports that often when she feels the need to urinate it comes on suddenly and is followed by an involuntary loss of urine. What is this condition termed?

a. Stress incontinence.
b. Bladder outlet obstruction.
c. Overflow incontinence.
d. Urge incontinence.

18) What is the commonest organism associated with urinary tract infection in the UK?

a. *Staphylococcus aureus*.
b. *Pseudomonas aeruginosa*.
c. *Escherichia coli*.
d. *Klebsiella spp.*

19) Where are staghorn calculi typically found?

a. In the renal pyramids.
b. In the renal pelvis.
c. As the ureter crosses the pelvic brim.
d. At the vesico-ureteric junction.

20) Failure to replace the foreskin after catheterisation may risk developing which of the following conditions?

a. Phimosis.
b. Balanitis xerotica obliterans.
c. Paraphimosis.
d. Urethral stricture.

21) What is the first-line management for suspected testicular torsion?

a. Ultrasound of testes with Doppler studies.
b. Urgent exploration of the scrotum within 6 hours of presentation.
c. Observe for 6 hours and offer surgery if the pain does not settle.
d. Urgent exploration of the scrotum within 6 hours of the onset of pain.

22) A young male has unilateral loin to groin pain and non-visible haematuria. What is the gold standard investigation?

a. CT of the urinary tract without contrast.
b. CT of the urinary tract with contrast.
c. X-ray of the urinary tract.
d. Ultrasound of the urinary tract.

23) Which of these factors is not associated with an increased risk of urinary tract infection?

a. Diabetes mellitus.
b. Renal tract stones.
c. Male gender.
d. Prostatic enlargement.

Extended matching questions

Disorders of the scrotum and testis

a. Hydrocele.
b. Varicocele.
c. Undescended testes.
d. Testicular torsion.

e. Epididymo-orchitis.
f. Testicular tumour.
g. Inguinal hernia.
h. Mumps orchitis.

Match the description of the patient with the most likely diagnosis.

1) A 63-year-old male with a tender scrotum with a dragging sensation that worsens after prolonged periods of standing. He describes his scrotum as feeling "like a bag of worms" to touch.

2) A 22-year-old male with severe and sudden unilateral testicular pain. He is unable to get comfortable and it is not relieved by painkillers. His right testis feels higher than usual.

3) A 19-year-old male with bilateral tender scrotal swelling. He has a temperature of 38.2°C and his face also appears bilaterally swollen.

4) A 43-year-old male with a unilateral painless scrotal swelling. It is not possible to get above the swelling and it transilluminates when a light is held to the skin.

5) A 25-year-old male with a gradual-onset unilateral testicular pain. A firm mass is palpable on examination which cannot be separated from the testis.

Management of haematuria

a. Routine outpatient review.
b. Urgent outpatient review.
c. Cystodiathermy.
d. Blood transfusion.

e. No investigation.
f. Three-way catheter and irrigation.
g. 12ch Foley catheter.
h. Repeat cystoscopy.

Match the description with the most appropriate management.

6) A 72-year-old male presents with episodes of painless visible haematuria. He is otherwise well in himself and his haemoglobin is 134g/L.

7) A 65-year-old male who takes warfarin and has known bladder cancer presents with acute urinary retention. He reports visible haematuria in the days beforehand but thought it would settle down if he stopped his warfarin. His INR is 1.6.

8) A 78-year-old male with known bladder cancer presents with haematuria. He looks pale and feels short of breath. His haemoglobin is 75g/L.

9) A 34-year-old male was catheterised for urinary retention while using epidural anaesthesia. He found the catheter insertion sore initially and had a small amount of visible haematuria but this stopped after a few hours and did not recur during his admission.

10) A 64-year-old female presents to the clinic with visible haematuria. She has had bladder cancer in the past but this was resected and her cystoscopy 11 months ago was clear. She is well in herself and her haemoglobin is 121g/L.

Disorders of the penis

a. Phimosis.

b. Paraphimosis.

c. Peyronie's disease.

d. Balanitis xerotica obliterans.

e. Penile fracture.

f. Hypospadias.

g. Squamous cell carcinoma.

h. Mondor's disease.

Match the description of the patient with the most likely diagnosis.

11) A 58-year-old male has noticed a well-demarcated ulcerated lesion on his glans. He does not report any trauma and sexual screening reveals no evidence of infection.

12) A 17-year-old complains of tightness of the foreskin when retracted. It has now become painful and swollen, and he is unable to return it to the original position.

13) A 65-year-old male has noticed tightness of the foreskin. He has well-circumscribed white patches on the glans and the skin appears dry.

14) A 42-year-old male complains of tightness of the foreskin. He has never been able to retract it fully but has not noticed any pain and he is still able to pass urine as usual.

15) A 34-year-old male reports that he has noticed a curvature in his penis when erect. He is unsure when it first started but it is getting worse and now intercourse is painful.

Lower urinary tract symptoms (LUTS)

a.   Benign prostatic enlargement.   e.   Bladder calculi.
b.   Overactive bladder.   f.   Transitional cell carcinoma.
c.   Side effect of medication.   g.   Prostatic adenocarcinoma.
d.   Urinary tract infection.   h.   Urethral stricture.

Match the description of the patient with the most likely diagnosis.

16)   A 23-year-old female presents with a 3-day history of frequency, urgency and dysuria. She has a normal stream. Urine dip is positive for nitrites and leucocytes.

17)   A 72-year-old male presents with increasing frequency, urgency and nocturia. He reports finding himself "wet" shortly after passing urine even though he feels he has finished.

18)   A 65-year-old male presents to the clinic with a long history of frequency, urgency and nocturia although his symptoms have improved with tamsulosin. He has recently had some haematuria and his primary care doctor found his PSA to be 8.1ng/L.

19)   A 44-year-old female presents with longstanding frequency and urgency of small amounts. She has no dysuria but has had some episodes of incontinence following urgency. The urine dip is negative.

20)   A 25-year-old male presents to the clinic with a difficulty passing urine. He has no frequency or dysuria but finds it difficult to initiate passing urine and has a poor stream when he does start. He was involved in a car accident earlier this year. His only medications are salbutamol inhalers and paracetamol when required.

Urinary tract infections

a.	Cystoscopy.	e.	CT scan of the renal tract.
b.	Oral antibiotics for 7-10 days.	f.	Intravenous antibiotics.
c.	Oral antibiotics for 3 days.	g.	Renal ultrasound.
d.	Surgical removal of stone.	h.	No treatment required.

Match the description of the patient with the most appropriate management.

21) A 45-year-old female has had recurrent infections with *Proteus mirabilis*. Pyelography shows a filling defect in the renal pelvis. Currently, she is well with no signs of active infection.

22) A 22-year-old female presents with frequency, urgency and dysuria. Her blood pressure is 118/83mmHg, heart rate is 76 beats per minute, temperature is 37.2°C. The urine dip is positive for leucocytes and nitrites.

23) A 36-year-old male has had three culture-proven urinary tract infections in the last 12 months. His antibiotics have been prescribed based on sensitivities and the infections have resolved each time. Currently he is well with no signs of active infection.

24) A 26-year-old female has a urine dip at her primary care doctor's practice to test for pregnancy. Her urine dip is negative for bHCG but is positive for leucocytes and nitrites. She reports no frequency or dysuria and feels well in herself.

25) A 31-year-old female presents with dysuria and flank pain. Her blood pressure is 87/56mmHg, heart rate is 114 beats per minute, temperature is 38.1°C and respiratory rate is 20 with an oxygen saturation of 97% on room air.

Paediatric urological conditions

a.	Retractile testis.	e.	Inguinal hernia.
b.	Paraphimosis.	f.	Hypospadias.
c.	Cryptorchidism.	g.	Hydrocele.
d.	Phimosis.	h.	Torsion.

Match the description of the patient with the most likely diagnosis.

26) A 2-year-old male has a tight foreskin that cannot be fully retracted. He is comfortable and able to pass urine without difficulty although his mother noticed once that the foreskin ballooned during urination.

27) A 6-week-old male undergoes a routine baby check. It is noted that the urethral opening is not present at the glans but opens on the distal shaft of the penis. He appears settled and comfortable.

28) A 14-year-old male presents with a unilateral acutely painful testicle. The pain radiates into his abdomen and he is unable to be comforted. There is no history of trauma.

29) A 4-month-old male is seen in the clinic with his father. At his routine baby checks it was noted that there was no testis palpable in the left hemiscrotum. The testis is still not palpable and his father reports it has been missing since birth.

30) An 18-month-old male has started to walk and his mother noticed he had a swollen right hemiscrotum on standing. The swelling is not seen when he lies down. On examination, the swelling transilluminates.

Management of disorders of the scrotum

a. Orchidectomy via an inguinal approach.
b. Orchidectomy via a scrotal approach.
c. Exploration of the scrotum.
d. Antibiotic treatment.
e. Scrotal support.
f. Surgical repair.
g. Ultrasound assessment.
h. No treatment required.

Match the description with the most appropriate management.

31) A 21-year-old male presents to the emergency department with a unilateral acutely painful testicle. The left testicle feels more horizontal than the right and is extremely tender on examination.

32) A 36-year-old male has a swollen scrotum that has been present for years. It does not usually cause him pain at rest but can feel cumbersome when he exercises. The swelling transilluminates. Ultrasound shows no testicular masses.

33) A 23-year-old male has been referred by his primary care doctor with a firm testicular lump. Imaging and tumour markers are highly suggestive of a malignancy.

34) A 24-year-old male has been referred to urology with a suspected testicular torsion. He has had unilateral testicular pain for 3 days. On examination, he has a tender testicle and epididymis but tolerates examination. There is no history of trauma.

35) A 56-year-old male has a swollen hemiscrotum on the left side. It has come on over the last few weeks and feels bumpy but soft and compressible. The swelling aches and increases over the course of the day but is relieved when he lies down.

Haematuria

a. Transitional cell carcinoma (TCC).   e.   Bladder stone.

b. Squamous cell carcinoma (SCC).   f.   Benign prostatic enlargement.

c. Renal cell carcinoma.   g.   Adenocarcinoma of the prostate.

d. Ureteric colic.   h.   Cystitis.

Match the description of the patient with the most likely diagnosis.

36) A 45-year-old Brazilian male presents to his primary care doctor with painless visible haematuria. He has no other medical conditions and is systemically well.

37) A 56-year-old male with multiple sclerosis has microscopic haematuria. He passes urine with manual pressure on the suprapubic area and has had recurrent urinary tract infections.

38) A 42-year-old male presents with flank pain and microscopic haematuria. He is unable to get comfortable but is systemically well.

39) A 59-year-old male presents with painless visible haematuria. He has worked as a painter and decorator for 40 years and smokes 20 cigarettes a day.

40) A 58-year-old male presents with visible haematuria. He has previously had rectal cancer which was treated with surgery and radiotherapy. He is systemically well but reports some frequency and dysuria. His urine dip is positive for blood and protein only.

Management of stone disease

a.   Analgesia and reassure.   e.   Ureteroscopic laser fragmentation.

b.   No treatment required.   f.   IV urogram.

c.   Antibiotics.   g.   CT KUB.

d.   Insertion of a JJ stent.   h.   Percutaneous nephrolithotomy.

Match the description with the most appropriate management.

41)   A 34-year-old male is unable to get comfortable with severe left-sided loin to groin pain and non-visible haematuria. He has never been diagnosed with renal stones in the past. He has some relief from morphine. His vital signs are: BP is 123/86mmHg, heart rate is 74, respiratory rate is 16, oxygen saturation is 96% on room air, temperature is 37.2°C.

42)   A 28-year-old male has a 4mm partially obstructing stone fragment in the left mid ureter. He has flank pain and vomiting. His vital signs are: BP is 85/64mmHg, heart rate is 95, respiratory rate is 20, oxygen saturation is 98% on room air, temperature is 38.4°C. He has already been given IV antibiotics and fluids.

43)   A 64-year-old female has a 24mm stone in the right renal pelvis. She has had recurrent urinary tract infections with some requiring hospitalisation. There is no evidence of active infection at present.

44)   A 31-year-old male presents to the emergency department with right flank pain radiating to the groin and one episode of pale visible haematuria. He is found to have a 3mm non-obstructing stone at the vesico-ureteric junction. His observations are stable and blood results are within normal parameters.

45)   A 44-year-old female with a previous history of stone disease is admitted with a 6mm partially obstructing stone in the left mid ureter. She is in severe pain with only mild relief from morphine and rectal diclofenac. Her vital signs are: BP is 121/84mmHg, heart rate is 70, respiratory rate is 16, oxygen saturation is 97% on room air, temperature is 37°C.

Short answer questions

1) A 55-year-old male presents to the emergency department with right-sided loin pain that radiates to his groin. It came on while at rest and he is unable to get comfortable. The junior doctor suspects this patient has renal colic.

a. What one other important diagnosis should be considered?   1 mark

b. Which investigation may confirm ureteric colic?   1 mark

c. State three common types of renal stones.   3 marks

d. Name three places where stones may cause urinary obstruction.   3 marks

e. Give one treatment option and an example of this.   2 marks

2) A 25-year-old female attends the emergency department with right-sided flank pain, vomiting and pyrexia. She reports urinary frequency and dysuria in the days prior to this.

a. What is the most likely diagnosis for this patient?   1 mark

b. What three investigations will help support this diagnosis?   3 marks

c. List two common symptoms of a urinary tract infection.   2 marks

d. List three factors that predispose to a urinary tract infection.   3 marks

e. Specify one treatment measure for a urinary tract infection.   1 mark

3) A 23-year-old male is referred by his primary care doctor with a testicular lump. He noticed it around 4 weeks ago and it feels hard and irregular.

a. State three ways this patient should be assessed. 3 marks

b. How are testicular tumours broadly classified? 1 mark

c. Testicular cancer typically metastasises via which route? 1 mark

d. Which two age groups are most affected by testicular cancer? 2 marks

e. State three ways a testicular tumour is usually managed. 3 marks

4) A 72-year-old male reports gradually increasing frequency of urine with nocturia and occasional post-micturition dribbling.

a. Explain how lower urinary tract symptoms are broadly divided and provide one example of each. 2 marks

b. What is the likely diagnosis for this patient? 1 mark

c. State two pharmacological treatments that are available. 2 marks

d. What is PSA and how is it relevant in this scenario? 2 marks

e. Name three common causes for bladder outlet obstruction. 3 marks

5) A 67-year-old retired factory worker has painless haematuria. He has smoked 20 cigarettes a day for 50 years.

a. State three ways this patient should be investigated. 3 marks

b. What are the two commonest types of bladder cancer? 1 mark

c. List two risk factors for bladder cancer. 2 marks

d. Describe three management options for bladder cancer. 3 marks

e. Explain how bladder cancer is staged. 1 mark

6) A 72-year-old male comes to the emergency department with abdominal pain. He has not passed urine for 24 hours despite the urge to go. A bladder scan shows >999ml in the bladder.

a. How should this patient be managed in the first instance? 1 mark
b. What might you find on examination? 1 mark
c. State three measures to manage this patient on the ward. 3 marks
d. List three causes of acute urinary retention. 3 marks
e. Should this patient be already known to have benign prostatic enlargement managed by medications, what is the next step? 2 marks

7) A 58-year-old male has an ultrasound scan for suspected gallstones. No evidence of gallstones is seen but there is an incidental finding of a renal mass on the left. The urine dipstick shows microscopic haematuria.

a. What is the most common type of tumour found in the kidney? 1 mark
b. State three symptoms a renal tumour typically presents with. 3 marks
c. Should a biopsy be taken? Explain your answer. 2 marks
d. How are renal tumours staged? 2 marks
e. What are the main options for management? 2 marks

8) A 22-year-old male presents to the emergency department with severe right-sided testicular pain. There is no history of trauma.

a. What diagnosis should be considered? 1 mark
b. State three features that would concern you on examination. 3 marks
c. State two measures to manage this patient. 2 marks
d. Name three important risks specific to the surgical management of this condition that should be discussed when gaining consent. 3 marks
e. What is the blood supply to the testicle? 1 mark

9) A 54-year-old male needs to be catheterised for a laparoscopic abdominal operation. His past medical history includes a pelvic fracture in his early twenties sustained during a car accident. The surgeon on call finds it difficult to pass the catheter and calls a urologist for help.

a. Given his past medical history what is the probable cause for the   1 mark
    difficulty passing a urinary catheter?
b. Define the three parts of the urethra.   3 marks
c. State the two main causes of urethral stricture.   2 marks
d. State two ways a urethral stricture may present.   2 marks
e. Name two management options for urethral structures.   2 marks

10) A 41-year-old female registers with a new primary care doctor and her screening urine dip is found to be positive for leucocytes and nitrites in urine. She has no urinary symptoms and feels well in herself with no comorbidities or medications.

a. Define bacteriuria.   1 mark
b. Define a urinary tract infection.   1 mark
c. Does this patient have a UTI? Explain your answer.   2 marks
d. Name the two commonest bacteria causing uncomplicated UTI.   2 marks
e. State four differences in the presentation of urinary tract infections 4 marks
    between children and the elderly.

11) A 68-year-old male is referred to the clinic with a PSA of 9.81ng/ml. He has been treated for LUTS with tamsulosin for several years with a satisfactory response but has no other urological history.

a.   What diagnosis would concern you?   1 mark

b.   How does prostate cancer typically grow and metastasise?   2 marks

c.   How is prostate cancer staged and graded?   2 marks

d.   How is PSA monitoring useful in management?   3 marks

e.   State two treatment options commonly used in prostate cancer.   2 marks

12) A 54-year-old male presents to the urology clinic with a swollen scrotum. It has been present for some time and is gradually increasing in size. His primary care doctor suspects a hydrocele so has referred him for further assessment.

a.   Name two features likely to be found on examination.   2 marks

b.   State two ways a hydrocele is usually managed.   2 marks

c.   What causes a congenital hydrocele?   1 mark

d.   What is a varicocele and how can this be distinguished from a hydrocele?   3 marks

e.   Why might a new-onset left varicocele be concerning?   2 marks

13) An 83-year-old male is catheterised for acute urinary retention. His admission blood results show a creatinine of 282μmol/L compared with 81μmol/L earlier in the month. Potassium and sodium are within normal parameters.

a.   How would you describe this biochemical picture?   1 mark

b.   How can this be classified by aetiology?   1.5 marks

c.   Give an example for each category.   1.5 marks

d.   How should the patient be managed in the case of these different aetiologies? 3 marks

e.   State three absolute indications for dialysis.   3 marks

Chapter 6

Neurosurgery
QUESTIONS

Single best answer questions

1) A patient arrives in the emergency department following a fall. He is opening his eyes to pain and is disorientated with confused speech but obeys commands. What is his GCS?

a. 5.
b. 8.
c. 10.
d. 12.

2) Which of the following is not part of the Cushing's reflex?

a. Hypertension.
b. Bradycardia.
c. Irregular respiration.
d. Tachycardia.

3) Which of the following does not indicate a possible base of skull fracture?

a.   Battle's sign (mastoid ecchymosis).
b.   Third cranial nerve palsy.
c.   Racoon eyes (periorbital ecchymosis).
d.   Halo sign.

4) Which of the following is an indication for an urgent CT of the head within 1 hour of admission?

a.   GCS less than 15, 2 hours after injury.
b.   GCS 13-15 at initial assessment.
c.   Feelings of nausea in adults.
d.   Haematoma formation without an obvious step.

5) What proportion of subarachnoid haemorrhages are caused by a ruptured berry aneurysm?

a.   60%.
b.   45%.
c.   85%.
d.   90%.

6) Which of the following is most often injured in an extradural haemorrhage?

a.   Accessory meningeal artery.
b.   Middle meningeal artery.
c.   Masseteric artery.
d.   Posterior deep temporal artery.

7) Which CT of the head finding is most consistent with an acute subdural haemorrhage?

a. Biconvex area of high density.
b. Hyperdense areas in the subarachnoid space.
c. Dilated ventricles bilaterally.
d. Crescentic hyperdense lesion on the inner surface of the skull.

8) Which imaging modality is most sensitive for bone involvement in space-occupying lesions?

a. CT.
b. MRI.
c. Angiography.
d. PET.

9) Which of the following is the most common type of primary CNS tumour?

a. Meningioma.
b. Lymphoma.
c. Glioma.
d. Medulloblastoma.

10) Which part of the optic tract is affected in bitemporal hemianopia?

a. Optic nerve.
b. Optic radiations.
c. Optic chiasm.
d. Lateral geniculate body.

11) Which of the following does not describe a high-grade tumour?

a. Likely malignant.
b. Aggressive.
c. Poorly differentiated.
d. Likely benign.

12) Which of the following conditions is often associated with bilateral vestibular schwannomas?

a. Neurofibromatosis 1.
b. Neurofibromatosis 2.
c. Tuberous sclerosis.
d. Arnold-Chiari malformation.

13) Which of the following is not a potential treatment of hydrocephalus?

a. Trans-sphenoidal surgery.
b. Furosemide and acetazolamide.
c. Lumbar puncture.
d. Ventriculoperitoneal shunt.

14) Which of the following corresponds to a score of M3 in the motor component on the GCS?

a. Obeys commands.
b. No response.
c. Extension in response to pain.
d. Flexion in response to pain.

15) During transfer to hospital a patient deteriorates and opens his eyes to voice. He is disorientated and confused when talking to him and he localises to painful stimuli. What is his GCS?

a. 11.
b. 12.
c. 13.
d. 14.

16) Which of the following is not an indication for a CT of the head within 1 hour of admission?

a. Suspected open or depressed skull fracture.
b. Two or more episodes of vomiting in adults.
c. Fall down more than 2 steps.
d. Focal neurological deficit.

17) Which of the following is not an aspect of general management of someone with a raised ICP?

a. Lie the patient flat to increase cerebral perfusion.
b. Normal or mild hypothermia.
c. Bed head raised to 30°.
d. Rapid treatment of seizures.

18) Below which GCS score do you worry about a patient being unable to safely maintain their own airway?

a. 10.
b. 8.
c. 14.
d. 9.

19) Which of the following features would you not expect to see on a CT of the head of an extradural haemorrhage?

a. Biconvex-shaped area of high density.
b. Midline shift.
c. Overlying soft tissue haematoma.
d. Blood in bilateral ventricles.

20) Which of these correctly defines an acute subdural haemorrhage?

a. 3-20 days.
b. >20 days.
c. <72 hours.
d. <7 days.

21) Which of the following is not an indication for a burr hole following a chronic subdural haemorrhage?

a. Symptomatic presentation.
b. Subdural haematoma present for >2 months.
c. Midline shift >5mm.
d. Haematoma >10mm.

22) Which of the following is not a hormone that could potentially be produced by a pituitary tumour?

a. Follicle-stimulating hormone.
b. Growth hormone.
c. Testosterone.
d. Luteinising hormone.

23) Which of the following symptoms is least likely to represent a vestibular schwannoma?

a.   Slurred speech.
b.   Hearing loss.
c.   Pressure sensation in the ear.
d.   Tinnitus.

Extended matching questions

Space-occupying lesion

a. Meningioma.

b. Intracranial abscess.

c. Tuberculoma.

d. Arachnoid cyst.

e. Glioma.

f. Pituitary tumour.

g. Cerebral metastases.

h. Vestibular schwannoma.

Match the patient presentation with the most likely diagnosis.

1) A 65-year-old female presents to the emergency department with a seizure and left-sided arm and leg weakness. She reports that this has become gradually worse over the last 3 months along with a headache which has become worse also. She has no significant past medical history.

2) A 45-year-old male presents to his primary care doctor complaining of hearing loss. He thought this was due to his age but he is concerned as it appears to only be on the right side. It has gradually worsened over the last 3 weeks and for the last 3 days he has had an almost constant "ringing" in the right ear also.

3) A 30-year-old male presents to the eye hospital with a 3-week history of visual changes. He has had gradually worsening sight and describes it as "tunnel vision"; he has gradually lost his peripheral vision. He also mentions some unusual discharge from his nipples which he is considering seeing his primary care doctor about.

4) A 40-year-old male with known lung cancer with bone metastases presents to the emergency department following a seizure. He has been having increasingly worsening headaches and nausea over the last 2 weeks but put these down to the side effects of chemotherapy.

5) A 35-year-old female of South Asian origin presents to her primary care doctor with headaches. Her headache is worse when waking in the morning and is worse on coughing. She has also had a fever and cough for the last 4 weeks, sometimes coughing up blood. Her chest X-ray demonstrates a circular shadow in the right upper lobe as well as multiple widespread small opacities throughout the lung fields. She is known to be HIV-positive.

Raised ICP

a. Idiopathic intracranial hypertension.

b. Glioma.

c. Subarachnoid haemorrhage.

d. Pituitary tumour.

e. Vestibular schwannoma.

f. Intracranial abscess.

g. Meningioma.

h. Hydrocephalus.

Match the description of the patient with the most likely diagnosis.

6) A 25-year-old female presents to the emergency department with a sudden-onset headache over her occiput which she describes as the "worst headache ever" and is associated with neck stiffness. She has a known medical history of polycystic kidney disease.

7) A 50-year-old male presents to the emergency department with worsening headaches. He had a subarachnoid haemorrhage 6 months ago and is very anxious that this has reoccurred. His family state he has also become more confused over recent weeks and has appeared unsteady on his feet. A CT of the head shows bilaterally dilated ventricles.

8) A 35-year-old female presents to her primary care doctor with recurrent headaches which are worst in the morning and exacerbated by coughing. She also mentions she occasionally has "halos" in her vision on bending over. She gave birth to a healthy baby boy 6 weeks previously; the pregnancy was uncomplicated. A CT of the head arranged by the doctor demonstrates normal sized ventricles and no other abnormality.

9) A 40-year-old male presents to his primary care doctor with a unilateral hearing loss and a feeling of fullness in his left ear. He has also felt nauseous for the last 2 weeks but has no other significant past medical history of note.

10) A 35-year-old female presents to her primary care doctor with gradually worsening right arm weakness and headaches. This has been ongoing for 3 weeks. The headaches are worse in the morning and are made worse by coughing.

Head injury

a.	Subdural haemorrhage.	e.	CVA.
b.	Subarachnoid haemorrhage.	f.	GCS 10.
c.	Extradural haemorrhage.	g.	GCS 11.
d.	Transient ischaemic attack.	h.	GCS 12.

Match the description of the patient with the most likely option.

11) A 54-year-old male presents to the emergency department with severe nausea and vomiting. He is known to alcohol services as a heavy drinker. His friend states he has been drowsy on and off for the last 3 weeks. On further questioning, he reports increasing headaches which sound like those associated with a raised ICP.

12) A 70-year-old female presents to the emergency department due to a period of right arm and leg weakness. This occurred out of the blue 6 hours ago and she had no warning. There is no evidence of a head injury. The symptoms lasted around 2 ½ hours and there were no other neurological sequelae. A neurological examination is completely normal.

13) A patient presents to the emergency department in a confused and drowsy state. She opens her eyes to voice, is making incomprehensible sounds and tries to grasp and remove painful stimuli. What is her GCS?

14) A 24-year-old rugby player attends the emergency department following a bad tackle. He sustained a bang to the side of his head and appeared to lose consciousness at the time momentarily. He now appears back to normal but as you are talking to him he becomes increasingly drowsy. You urgently arrange a CT scan of his head.

15) A male is brought into the emergency department following a motorbike accident. He is confused and disorientated when you see him, his eyes open spontaneously and he withdraws in response to painful stimuli. What is his GCS at this time?

CT head

a. Subarachnoid haemorrhage.
b. Subdural haemorrhage.
c. Extradural haemorrhage.
d. Idiopathic intracranial hypertension.

e. Cerebral metastasis.
f. Meningioma.
g. Intracranial abscess.
h. Hydrocephalus.

Match the presentation and CT scan to the most likely diagnosis.

16) A 34-year-old female presents with a severe headache of sudden onset. A CT of the head demonstrates a hyperdense area in the subarachnoid space with blood between the ventricles.

17) A 35-year-old female presents with a persistent headache for 4 weeks. It has been worse in the mornings or last thing at night and she has experienced associated nausea. A CT of the head, however, shows no abnormality with normal appearances of brain parenchyma and normal ventricles.

18) A 20-year-old presents following a fall and head injury. The patient lost consciousness for around 2 minutes following the head injury and appeared back to their normal self on arrival. A CT of the head shows a biconcave area of high density (lens shape) underlying the site of impact.

19) A 65-year-old female presents following a fall. She has had a persistent headache since the fall and also shows some signs of altered neurology. A CT of the head demonstrates a crescent-shaped lesion and some midline shift.

20) A 70-year-old male presents to the emergency department as his family are concerned about him. For the last few weeks he has been increasingly confused and unsteady on his feet. He has also had a couple of episodes of urinary incontinence. A CT of the head shows enlarged ventricles bilaterally but nothing else of note.

Management options

a.	Subarachnoid haemorrhage.	e.	Cerebral metastasis.
b.	Subdural haemorrhage.	f.	Meningioma.
c.	Extradural haemorrhage.	g.	Intracranial abscess.
d.	Idiopathic intracranial hypertension.	h.	Hydrocephalus.

Match the management options with the most likely diagnosis.

21) Pre-operative corticosteroids and anti-epileptic medications.

22) Fluid resuscitation to avoid cerebral hypotension and a vessel clip or coiling by interventional radiology.

23) Surgical evacuation of haematoma of a biconcave bleed.

24) Furosemide and acetazolamide.

25) Repeated lumbar punctures.

Head injury

a.	GCS 7.	e.	GCS 11.
b.	GCS 3.	f.	GCS 9.
c.	GCS 5.	g.	GCS 15.
d.	GCS 6.	h.	GCS 12.

Match the description with the correct Glasgow Coma Scale score.

26) A young female presents in status epilepticus. When this has resolved using IV management, she opens her eyes to painful stimuli, does not make any vocal effort or sounds and withdraws to pain.

27) A male patient presents to the emergency department in DKA. He becomes increasingly drowsy until his eyes do not open to any stimuli, he is making incomprehensible sounds and he has abnormal flexion to pain.

28) A patient presents to the emergency department having been found in the street unresponsive. Upon arrival, they open their eyes in response to voice, are making incomprehensible sounds and withdraw to painful stimuli.

29) A patient collapses whilst waiting for a primary care doctor appointment. The doctor is talking to the ambulance crew and describes the patient as opening their eyes spontaneously, using inappropriate words and localising to pain.

30) A patient collapses whilst waiting to be seen in the emergency department. They are not opening their eyes to any stimuli, are making no vocal effort and are making no motor response whatsoever.

Glasgow Coma Scale

a. GCS 3.   e. GCS 5.
b. GCS 14.   f. GCS 12.
c. GCS 8.   g. GCS 2.
d. GCS 15.   h. GCS 6.

Match the description with the correct Glasgow Coma Scale score.

31) A 38-year-old cyclist is involved in a road traffic accident and his helmet is broken. On arrival to the emergency department he has his eyes open, is talking to staff, knows where he is, and is able to carry out the tasks you describe.

32) The same cyclist then deteriorates. He opens his eyes only when painful stimuli are applied. The patient does not remember being in hospital and thinks he is in the supermarket. He is still able to lift his arms when you ask him.

33) The cyclist then deteriorates further. He is still responding to pain but not voice. He is making strange noises which don't seem to be words and he is extending in response to pain.

34) The cyclist is transferred to the CT scanner but on the way he stops responding to pain. He is not making any sound and makes no movement to pain or to commands.

35) Following emergency neurosurgery the cyclist is in recovery. He is sat up in bed, looking around the room. He is talking to the nursing staff but is not aware where he is at present. He is able to lift his arms when requested.

Raised intracranial pressure

a. Subarachnoid haemorrhage.
b. Pituitary tumour.
c. Idiopathic intracranial hypertension.
d. Vestibular schwannoma.

e. Intracranial abscess.
f. Hydrocephalus.
g. Meningioma.
h. Tuberculoma.

Match the description of the patient with the most likely diagnosis.

36) A young male presents to the emergency department with "the worst headache ever". He was on a run when it suddenly hit, he has vomited numerous times and has severe neck stiffness.

37) A 35-year-old female presents to her primary care doctor complaining of having missed her last 3 periods. She has been trying for a baby recently but all pregnancy tests are negative so far. She has also had a headache persistently but has so far put this down to the stress of her situation. It is worse in the mornings and on straining to go to the toilet.

38) A 34-year-old female presents to the emergency department 5 weeks postpartum complaining of a severe headache, worse in the morning and on coughing. She has no other focal neurology. On retinal examination, she has what you think is papilloedema but conversely the CT of the head is normal.

39) A 60-year-old male is admitted to the emergency department following a seizure. He had a single, isolated seizure that lasted for 2 minutes. His family report he has had some numbness and tingling in his left arm, worsening progressively for the preceding 2 months.

40) A 40-year-old male sees his primary care doctor for ongoing buzzing in both his ears. He has had some reduction in his hearing also. The doctor also notes some light brown spots in the patient's armpits which the patient states were spotted at birth but then he has moved around a lot and not followed these up.

Space-occupying lesion

a.	Meningioma.	e.	Arachnoid cyst.
b.	Pituitary tumour.	f.	Vestibular schwannoma.
c.	Cerebral metastases.	g.	Tuberculoma.
d.	Intracranial abscess.	h.	Haematoma.

Match the description of the patient with the most likely diagnosis.

41) A 32-year-old male presents to the emergency department with fever, rigors and sweats. He has had severe headaches recently which are improved by standing. He is a known IV drug user. His chest X-ray looks normal and there is a well-circumscribed lesion present on a contrast CT of the head.

42) A 95-year-old female presents to the emergency department with a reduced GCS. She fell over at home last night where she hit her head and has had a severe, worsening headache since then. She is on warfarin for AF and has not had her INR checked for a week as she has been away on holiday.

43) A 60-year-old female presents with severe headaches to her primary care doctor. She is currently undergoing chemotherapy following a successful resection of a primary lung tumour and some lymph nodes. The headaches are worse in the mornings and late evening, and improved on standing. A CT of the head demonstrates multiple small lesions throughout the cerebrum.

44) A 40-year-old male presents to his primary care doctor with visual symptoms. He has noticed a gradual worsening of vision in his right visual field over the last few weeks. He has also been getting gradually worsening headaches for the same amount of time. He has no known past medical history and no other neurological signs or symptoms.

45) A 25-year-old male presents to his primary care doctor with a 2-month history of ringing in his left ear and severe left-sided facial pain. This is much worse when he chews or smiles. He has also noticed his hearing reduced in his left ear compared with normal.

Short answer questions

1) A 34-year-old male attends the emergency department with severe headaches when waking in the morning, made worse on coughing. He has a background of meningitis but has been well apart from the headaches for the last few years. He also states he feels slightly unsteady on walking. The doctor who sees him is concerned about hydrocephalus.

a.   What would you expect to see on a CT of the head?   2 marks
b.   Name two other symptoms you might see.   2 marks
c.   Which cranial nerve is most often affected?   2 marks
d.   Name two potential causes of hydrocephalus.   2 marks
e.   Name one medical and one surgical management option.   2 marks

2) A 26-year-old male is brought into the emergency department following a bicycle accident. He was hit by a car and his helmet is in several pieces on the trolley. He is opening his eyes in response to pain, is making noises which do not appear to be words and is flexing abnormally in response to pain. Whilst in resus he becomes markedly hypertensive and his pulse rate falls.

a.   Calculate this patient's GCS score.   1 mark
b.   What is the reflex he is exhibiting with the high BP and low pulse rate? 2 marks
c.   What would you expect to happen next in this reflex?   2 marks
d.   What is the overall cause of this reflex?   2 marks
e.   Name three important aspects of management in this case.   3 marks

3) A 34-year-old male is attacked on a night out with friends. He was kicked in the head repeatedly. He has a GCS of 7/15. He has bruising appearing behind both ears as he is wheeled into resus. On examination, you feel a step over one of the areas of injury on the parietal region of his head with a surrounding haematoma.

a. What is the name of the sign described above?   2 marks
b. Name two other features that might imply brain injury or a base of   2 marks
   skull fracture.
c. Given this patient's GCS, what is a main priority?   1 mark
d. What do you think is the most likely cause for the 'step' felt on   2 marks
   examination?
e. Apart from a CT of the head, name and describe one other method of   3 marks
   searching for CSF leakage.

4) A 56-year-old female presents to the emergency department following a seizure. She is not known to be epileptic and has not previously had seizures. She has had progressively worsening numbness in her left arm for the preceding 4 weeks and occasional but worsening headaches. You are concerned that she may have a space-occupying lesion.

a. What is the most common primary CNS tumour in adults?   2 marks
b. Where is this patient's tumour most likely to be located?   2 marks
c. Name two conditions these tumours can be associated with.   2 marks
d. Which imaging modality would be best to assess for tumour or   1 mark
   oedema involvement?
e. Tumours can be categorised as high or low grade. What is meant by   3 marks
   tumour grade?

5) An elderly female presents to her primary care doctor complaining of a unilateral hearing loss in her right ear. She has no other symptoms at this time. The doctor is concerned that it is a vestibular schwannoma.

a. What is a vestibular schwannoma? 2 marks
b. State one condition these can be associated with. 1 mark
c. Name three other signs or symptoms you may see in this patient. 3 marks
d. What management would you choose for this patient? 2 marks
e. Name two possible complications of surgical management. 2 marks

6) A 40-year-old female presents to the emergency department with an acute-onset headache. She states this is worse first thing in the morning and improves on standing up. On examination, it is noted she has what is thought to be bilateral papilloedema. A CT scan indicates hydrocephalus.

a. What would you expect to see on a CT scan of someone with hydrocephalus? 1 marks
b. List three other signs or symptoms for hydrocephalus. 3 marks
c. What are the two different types of hydrocephalus? 2 marks
d. Name two potential causes of hydrocephalus. 2 marks
e. State one medical and one surgical management for hydrocephalus. 2 marks

7) A 42-year-old female attends the emergency department with a severe headache. This suddenly started about 3 hours ago and was like she was hit over the back of the head. It is associated with vomiting, nausea and neck stiffness. Her only past medical history is a kidney problem but she is unsure what this is. You are concerned about a subarachnoid haemorrhage (SAH) and arrange an urgent CT of the head.

a. What is the most common cause of SAH? | 2 marks
b. State three findings on a CT of the head for a patient with SAH. | 3 marks
c. What two management steps can be initiated at the bedside? | 2 marks
d. Name one definitive management step for treating SAH. | 1 mark
e. Name two potential complications of SAH. | 2 marks

8) A 25-year-old rugby player is brought into the emergency department following a head injury during a match. He seems well now but you have previously read about these types of cases and know they are at risk of an extradural haemorrhage.

a. Which bone is often injured in an extradural haemorrhage? | 1 mark
b. Which artery is often damaged in an extradural haemorrhage? | 2 marks
c. What is the classically described course for these patients? | 3 marks
d. State two CT head findings for extradural haemorrhage. | 2 marks
e. Name two definitive treatment options. | 2 marks

9) An elderly female is brought into the emergency department because her family are concerned about her since she fell and hit the left side of her head a few days previously. She has been complaining of a headache and has been drowsy on and off since the head injury. On examination, her left pupil looks larger than the right. You are concerned about a subdural haemorrhage (SDH).

a. Which vessels are often affected in subdural haematoma? 2 marks

b. What might explain the dilated left pupil above? 3 marks

c. State two findings on a CT of the head for a patient with SDH. 2 marks

d. How would the CT appearance change in chronic SDH? 2 marks

e. Name one step in the management of acute SDH. 1 mark

10) A 34-year-old female presents to her primary care doctor with headaches and amenorrhoea. The headaches are worse in the morning and improved on standing. She has also noticed her peripheral vision is slowly deteriorating. Her doctor is worried about a pituitary tumour.

a. Oversecretion of which hormone is most likely to be causing this patient's amenorrhoea? 1 mark

b. What is the medical term for her visual symptoms? 2 marks

c. What is causing this visual change? 2 marks

d. Name three hormones you would test for in this patient. 3 marks

e. State two complications of resection of the pituitary gland. 2 marks

11) A cyclist is knocked off his bike by a lorry and he suffers a head injury. He is opening his eyes to speech, appears disorientated and is able to follow commands. He becomes profoundly hypertensive and bradycardic. You suspect his intracranial pressure is elevated.

a. What is this patient's GCS? — 1 mark
b. What is shown by the hypertension and bradycardia? — 2 marks
c. What is a normal intracranial pressure? — 2 marks
d. Which two pressures determine cerebral perfusion pressure? — 2 marks
e. Name three aspects of general management of a raised ICP. — 3 marks

12) A 57-year-old male is found unconscious in the park. On arrival to the emergency department, he is not responding to voice, making no sounds whatsoever and when painful stimuli are applied he abnormally flexes his limbs.

a. What is this patient's GCS? — 1 mark
b. What is the term for the abnormal flexion to pain? — 2 marks
c. List two investigations for this patient. — 2 marks
d. His GCS is below 8. What is a main priority at this time? — 2 marks
e. Name three complications of a long period coma. — 3 marks

13) A 15-year-old is brought to the emergency department following a fall from 10 feet causing a head injury. He has a large haematoma over the right side of his head and some bruising behind the ears as well as bilateral black eyes.

a. What is the term used for bruising behind the ears? — 1 mark
b. What is the term used for bilateral black eyes? — 1 mark
c. What is the major concern raised by the two above signs? — 2 marks
d. Name four bones in the skull that are more at risk of fracture. — 4 marks
e. State two other signs of a base of skull fracture. — 2 marks

Chapter 7

ENT surgery
QUESTIONS

Single best answer questions

1) What is the first-line treatment for acute otitis media?

a. Amoxicillin.
b. Ciprofloxacin.
c. Otomize spray.
d. Watch and wait.

2) Which salivary glands are the most common site for sialolithiasis?

a. Lingual.
b. Parotid.
c. Sublingual.
d. Submandibular.

3) What is the most common organism causing epiglottitis?

a. *Haemophilus influenzae*.
b. *Mycoplasma pneumoniae*.
c. Respiratory syncytial virus.
d. *Streptococcus pneumoniae*.

4)   Which of these examination findings suggest a conductive hearing loss in the right ear?

a.   Rinne's test negative both ears, Weber's test equal both ears.
b.   Rinne's test negative left ear, Weber's test lateralises to left.
c.   Rinne's test negative right ear, Weber's test lateralises to left.
d.   Rinne's test negative right ear, Weber's test lateralises to right.

5)   How should a pinna haematoma be managed?

a.   Aspiration or incision and drainage as soon as possible.
b.   Conservative management.
c.   Leave for 48 hours to allow inflammation to settle, then aspiration.
d.   Topical antibiotics.

6)   When should nasal packs be used for a patient with epistaxis?

a.   If a Foley catheter has been unsuccessful in stopping the bleeding.
b.   If first aid and cautery have been unsuccessful.
c.   In all patients on anticoagulation.
d.   In hypertensive patients.

7)   Which of these patient groups has a higher incidence of otitis media with effusion?

a.   Down's syndrome.
b.   Edwards' syndrome.
c.   Fragile X syndrome.
d.   Turner's syndrome.

8) What condition would an 'attic crust' suggest?

a. Acute otitis media.
b. Cholesteatoma.
c. Mastoiditis.
d. Otosclerosis.

9) How is otosclerosis inherited?

a. Autosomal dominant.
b. Autosomal recessive.
c. Mitochondrial.
d. X-linked.

10) Where is the most common site for ectopic thyroid tissue?

a. Base of the tongue.
b. Hyoid bone.
c. Pharynx.
d. Thyroglossal duct.

11) Which of these is part of Samter's triad?

a. Enlargement of the adenoids.
b. Eustachian tube dysfunction.
c. Nasal congestion.
d. Nasal polyps.

12) Which of these is a sign of otitis media with effusion?

a. Bulging tympanic membrane.
b. Dull tympanic membrane.
c. Ear pain.
d. Sensorineural hearing loss.

13) Where does the Eustachian tube open?

a. Hypopharynx.
b. Laryngopharynx.
c. Nasopharynx.
d. Oropharynx.

14) Which of these is not a risk factor for laryngeal carcinoma?

a. Epstein-Barr virus.
b. *Herpes simplex* virus.
c. Human immunodeficiency virus.
d. Human papilloma virus.

15) What is the first-line investigation for an ingested foreign body?

a. CT abdomen.
b. CT chest.
c. Lateral neck and chest X-rays.
d. MRI neck and chest.

16) What is the most common cause of epistaxis?

a. Anticoagulation.
b. Clotting disorders.
c. Old age.
d. Trauma.

17) Which two cranial nerves supply sensation to the pinna, along with branches of the cervical plexus?

a. Facial and trigeminal.
b. Facial and vagal.
c. Trigeminal and vagal.
d. Trigeminal and vestibulocochlear.

18) What is the most common histology in laryngeal cancers?

a. Adenocarcinoma.
b. Carcinoid tumour.
c. Lymphoma.
d. Squamous cell carcinoma.

19) Which examination finding of a neck lump would suggest a thyroglossal cyst?

a. Firm to palpate.
b. Located to the left of the midline.
c. Moves on protruding the tongue.
d. Moves on swallowing.

20) What investigation should be done for an adult with otitis media with effusion?

a. Ear swab.
b. Nasendoscopy.
c. None.
d. Tympanogram.

21) When should a cystic hygroma be removed surgically?

a. Always.
b. If it is affecting the function of adjacent structures.
c. If it is over 5cm in diameter.
d. Never.

22) What is the nerve supply to the vocal cords?

a. External laryngeal nerve.
b. Glossopharyngeal nerve.
c. Internal laryngeal nerve.
d. Recurrent laryngeal nerve.

23) Which of these features is most suggestive of benign paroxysmal positional vertigo?

a. Deafness.
b. Nystagmus.
c. Painful ears.
d. Tinnitus.

Extended matching questions

Ear pain

a. Acute otitis media.
b. Ear trauma.
c. Foreign body.
d. Mastoiditis.

e. Nasopharyngeal tumour.
f. Otitis externa.
g. Ramsay-Hunt syndrome.
h. Stroke.

Match the description of the patient with the most likely diagnosis.

1) A 52-year-old female presents with a painful right ear, associated with a rash on the pinna. She is very worried because she is unable to move the right side of her face.

2) A 4-year-old male visits his primary care doctor with left ear pain and says he can hear buzzing.

3) A 15-year-old female sees the nurse practitioner with yellow discharge and severe pain in her right ear.

4) A 67-year-old male from Beijing is visiting his daughter in the UK when he develops recurrent nosebleeds. He has also had a dull ache in his right ear for the last month.

5) A 7-year-old male presents with pain and discharge from his left ear. He is given a course of amoxicillin but comes back to the primary care doctor because he is no better and his aunt has noticed that his ear is sticking out more than the right one.

Sore throat

a.	Deep neck space infection.	e.	Laryngeal carcinoma.
b.	Food bolus.	f.	Pharyngitis.
c.	Ingested foreign body.	g.	Quinsy.
d.	Infectious mononucleosis.	h.	Tonsillitis.

Match the description of the patient with the most likely diagnosis.

6) A 15-year-old male sees his primary care doctor with a sore throat and feeling generally unwell. He is prescribed a course of amoxicillin and is advised to stay hydrated. The next day he comes back with a red rash all over his body.

7) A 40-year-old female has a sore throat and runny nose. On examination, her throat looks pink, her tonsils are not enlarged and her temperature is 37.2°C.

8) A 33-year-old plumber presents to the emergency department with severe throat pain. She is drooling and on examination there is swelling on the left side of her throat. Her uvula is deviated to the right.

9) A 56-year-old farmer has been celebrating his wife's birthday by finishing off the mixed grill at their local pub. He arrives at the emergency department soon after the meal very angry and red in the face, pointing at his throat and complaining of the worst pain in his life.

10) A 38-year-old male taking etanercept for ankylosing spondylitis collapses in the street. His friend tells the paramedics he has been complaining of a sore throat and a stiff neck for the last 2 days.

Neck lumps

a. Branchial cyst.
b. Cystic hygroma.
c. Dermoid cyst.
d. Lymphoma.

e. Reactive lymph node.
f. Salivary gland tumour.
g. Thyroglossal cyst.
h. Thyroid adenoma.

Match the description of the patient with the most likely diagnosis.

11) A 60-year-old female notices a lump at the front of her neck. It moves up and down when she swallows.

12) A 22-year-old male visits the walk-in centre with a lump in the right side of his neck which has been present for 4 days. On examination, it is mobile and soft and is approximately 1cm in diameter.

13) The health visitor notes that a 2-year-old child has a lump posterior to the sternocleidomastoid on the left side. The lump is soft and not painful.

14) A 33-year-old female sees the primary care doctor with a sore throat. She has several small lumps in her neck and under her chin. She is feeling hot.

15) A 57-year-old female sees the primary care doctor because she has started sweating at night again after finishing HRT. She has several small lumps in her neck and under her chin.

Hearing loss

a. Acoustic neuroma.
b. Cholesteatoma.
c. Cefuroxime.
d. Gentamicin.

e. Menière's disease.
f. Otitis media with effusion.
g. Otosclerosis.
h. Presbycusis.

Match the description of the patient with the most likely diagnosis.

16) A baby is found to have sensorineural hearing loss on her newborn hearing screen. During pregnancy her mother was admitted with an infection and given antibiotics.

17) A 54-year-old male is brought to the emergency department because he fell over on an escalator. He mentions that he has noticed hearing loss in his right ear over the past few weeks.

18) A 40-year-old female sees her primary care doctor because her husband has complained she is turning the TV up to astronomical levels. Her mother wears hearing aids.

19) A 37-year-old sous chef has had several ear infections in the last year. He comes to see his primary care doctor because he feels he can't hear as well in his right ear. On examination, the tympanic membrane looks retracted and the doctor notices a brown flake superiorly.

20) A 92-year-old male frequently needs things to be repeated for him loudly. He is otherwise well and is not too upset as he finds small talk tedious.

Swallowing problems

a.	Food bolus.	e.	Oesophageal carcinoma.
b.	Epiglottitis.	f.	Pharyngeal carcinoma.
c.	Globus hystericus.	g.	Stroke.
d.	Ingested foreign body.	h.	Quinsy.

Match the description of the patient with the most likely diagnosis.

21) A 5-year-old girl is brought to the emergency department by her father. She is distressed and drooling and her breathing sounds are abnormal and high-pitched.

22) A 62-year-old male presents with dysphagia and ear pain on the right.

23) A 10-year-old male with an autistic spectrum disorder is brought to the primary care doctor because he has started screaming and pointing to his chest during a meal.

24) A 44-year-old female comes to the emergency department with a feeling of a lump in her throat and difficulty swallowing. A chest X-ray and bloods are normal.

25) A 4-year-old girl is brought to the emergency department in an ambulance after having a seizure. Her family is very wealthy and have recently moved into a large suburban house built in 1884, which they have started redecorating. She is given some crisps when she recovers but regurgitates them and cries that she has pain in her chest.

Dizziness

a.   Acoustic neuroma.
b.   Benign paroxysmal positional vertigo.
c.   Otitis media.
d.   Menière's disease.

e.   Migraine.
f.   Postural hypotension.
g.   Stroke.
h.   Vestibular neuritis.

Match the description of the patient with the most likely diagnosis.

26)   A 64-year-old male has noticed that the room starts spinning whenever he stands up over the last month. He has a buzzing noise in his left ear.

27)   A 45-year-old cruise ship entertainer has a several-year history of attacks of vertigo every 2 months. During the attacks she is unable to work as she cannot cope with the movement of the ship. Examination is normal.

28)   A 38-year-old hairdresser complains that he feels like the room is spinning, especially in bed. On examination, he has rotational nystagmus on turning his head.

29)   A 29-year-old female calls her primary care doctor because she cannot get out of bed due to dizziness. She has also been vomiting since the middle of the night.

30)   A 76-year-old diabetic female has a sudden onset of vertigo while shopping for a new TV.

Airway management

a.	Adrenaline IM.	e.	IV antibiotics.
b.	Cardiopulmonary resuscitation.	f.	Open the wound.
c.	Cricothyroidotomy.	g.	Oral steroids.
d.	Intubate.	h.	Tracheostomy.

Choose the best first-line management for each airway issue.

31) A 5-year-old boy arrives in the emergency department with stridor. He appears distressed and is drooling. He moved to the UK 4 months ago and has not had any childhood vaccinations.

32) A 32-year-old female has had a total thyroidectomy earlier in the day for Graves' disease. The junior doctor is called to see her because her saturations are dropping. Her neck diameter has increased by 2cm.

33) A 17-year-old girl is admitted to hospital with tonsillitis because she cannot swallow fluids. She is treated with phenoxymethylpenicillin. The nurses ask for her to be seen as she complains of feeling very unwell. On examination, her skin is blotchy, her lips are swollen and her respiratory rate is 40.

34) A 72-year-old male has been diagnosed with laryngeal cancer. He arrives in the emergency department in respiratory distress and is unable to talk to tell the doctors what has happened.

35) A 55-year-old restaurant critic is feasting on tuna steak in a new gastropub. He suddenly starts coughing and pointing to his neck. The waiter tries to help him by giving backslaps but he collapses to the floor. The waiter cannot hear or see any signs of breathing.

Ear discharge

a.	Barotrauma.	e.	Mastoiditis.
b.	Cholesteatoma.	f.	Otitis externa.
c.	CSF leak.	g.	Otitis media.
d.	Malignant otitis externa.	h.	Psoriasis.

Match the description of the patient with the most likely diagnosis.

36) A 28-year-old male presents to his primary care doctor 5 days after returning from a holiday where he had been swimming a lot. He has pain and discharge from his right ear. On examination, the ear canal is erythematous and discharge is noted. Pain is increased by pressing on the tragus. The tympanic membrane looks normal.

37) A 30-year-old diving instructor notices discharge from her left ear and a whistling sound when she blows her nose.

38) A 6-year-old girl has pain and discharge from her right ear which has been present for 2 days.

39) A 45-year-old female sees her primary care doctor with aching in her right ear and foul-smelling discharge. She has had three courses of antibiotics for ear infections in the last year but says this is less painful than those infections.

40) A 61-year-old diabetic male comes to the emergency department because he is having very severe pain in his left ear with large amounts of discharge. He is also having headaches on the right side and feels generally unwell.

Change in voice

a.   Acromegaly.   e.   Lung cancer.
b.   Bulbar palsy.   f.   Stroke.
c.   Laryngeal cancer.   g.   Surgery.
d.   Laryngitis.   h.   Vocal nodules.

Match the description of the patient with the most likely diagnosis.

41)   A 54-year-old opera singer speaks to her vocal coach as she has noticed that her voice has gradually become more hoarse and breathy. She feels otherwise well.

42)   A 64-year-old smoker is referred to ENT because his voice sounds hoarse. He has lost 6kg over the last 2 months. On flexible nasendoscopy, his vocal cords do not fully appose. No masses are visualised.

43)   A 47-year-old female has recently been treated for Graves' disease. She complains that her voice is much quieter than it was before.

44)   An 18-year-old student goes to the walk-in centre as he has a hoarse voice and sore throat.

45)   An 80-year-old male is brought to hospital by his daughter as he has woken up with slurred speech.

Short answer questions

1) A 78-year-old female is on the cardiology ward as she has developed AF. She has a background of Alzheimer's disease and currently has a cold. She has been started on warfarin to decrease her stroke risk. The junior doctor is called to see her as she has developed a nose bleed.

a.	Name two risk factors for this patient developing epistaxis.	2 marks
b.	What anatomical area do most nose bleeds originate from?	1 mark
c.	State four ways that this patient should initially be managed.	4 marks
d.	Name two treatments if initial measures do not stop the bleeding.	2 marks
e.	Name one possible complication of epistaxis.	1 mark

2) A 7-year-old male is seen by his primary care doctor as he has been having trouble in lessons at school. He has been missing things the teacher has said and not concentrating. The doctor examines him and suspects otitis media with effusion (OME).

a.	Name two signs of OME on examination.	2 marks
b.	State one investigation that should be requested.	1 mark
c.	Name one condition that may predispose a child to OME.	1 mark
d.	Name two non-surgical and one surgical treatment options.	3 marks
e.	Give three possible problems caused by non-resolving OME.	3 marks

3) A 56-year-old lawyer presents to his primary care doctor as he has noticed a change in his voice over the last 2 weeks and says he sounds hoarser than before. On further questioning, the doctor finds that he has lost half a stone this month, without trying to diet. The doctor is concerned the patient may have cancer and refers him onto a 2-week wait pathway.

a. Name three risk factors for head and neck cancer.   3 marks
b. State one investigation to perform prior to referral.   1 mark
c. The patient is found to have a T2 N1 M0 laryngeal tumour. What will   2 marks
   his surgery have to include for a chance of a cure?
d. The patient has his operation and is treated with adjuvant   1 mark
   radiotherapy. Define "adjuvant".
e. State three complications that may arise from his surgery.   3 marks

4) A 37-year-old office worker visits her primary care doctor because she has been having attacks of vertigo at work. The doctor asks her about any other symptoms and finds that she has also noticed ringing in her ears and feels as if her ears are blocked. The doctor refers her to ENT and she is diagnosed with Menière's disease.

a. State one investigation to help diagnosis Menière's disease.   1 mark
b. What pathological change is usually seen in the ears?   1 mark
c. Name two treatments that can be used to treat this disease.   2 marks
d. What three treatments are given for vertigo in Menière's disease?   3 marks
e. State three treatments used for hearing loss in Menière's disease.   3 marks

5) A 29-year-old teaching assistant presents to the primary care doctor with a 24-hour history of right ear pain and discharge. On examination, the tympanic membrane is reddened and bulging. Her temperature is 36.8°C and other observations are normal. The doctor treats as for acute otitis media.

a.	Name two possible causative organisms.	2 marks
b.	Give two risk factors for developing acute otitis media.	2 marks
c.	Name three treatment options for this patient.	3 marks
d.	Name one complication from acute otitis media.	1 mark
e.	State two features to suggest a patient needs hospital admission.	2 marks

6) A 49-year-old female has noticed a swelling beneath her chin. It becomes painful when she eats. Her doctor tells her that she probably has a stone in her salivary duct.

a.	Name the three main salivary glands.	3 marks
b.	Name one investigation to confirm the diagnosis.	1 mark
c.	State two medical and one surgical methods to manage a salivary duct calculus.	3 marks
d.	Name two other causes of salivary gland inflammation.	2 marks
e.	Give one complication of salivary gland inflammation.	1 mark

7) A 22-year-old student visits her primary care doctor with a severe sore throat. The doctor is worried she may have a quinsy and refers her to the ENT emergency clinic.

a.	Give two features that would suggest a quinsy on examination.	2 marks
b.	Name four medical management options.	4 marks
c.	What is the definitive management of this condition?	1 mark
d.	What is the most common causative organism?	1 mark
e.	Give two complications if a quinsy is left untreated.	2 marks

8) A 72-year-old male is referred to ENT because he has noticed a swelling in front of his right ear which has been present for about 4 weeks. The swelling is not painful and he feels otherwise well.

a. Name two features on examination to suggest malignancy.   2 marks
b. State two investigations that should be performed.   2 marks
c. The patient decides he does not want any investigation and would like   1 mark
   to watch and wait. He comes back to clinic 4 weeks later and has
   developed a right-sided facial droop. What is the most likely histology
   of his tumour?
d. State four complications that may arise from surgery.   4 marks
e. What would the treatment be for a benign parotid tumour?   1 mark

9) A 33-year-old prisoner is brought to the emergency department having been involved in a fight where he was knocked out after refusing to share his contraband cigarettes. He undergoes a primary survey and stabilisation and is found to have mainly facial injuries as well as fractured ribs.

a. What investigation is needed prior to managing facial injuries?   1 mark
b. On examination, the patient's nose appears deformed. When looking   2 marks
   inside the nose the septum looks swollen in both nostrils and appears
   purplish in colour. What has caused this appearance and how should
   it be managed?
c. The patient has a nasal fracture. State three management options for   3 marks
   this patient.
d. Later that evening the junior doctor is called to see the patient   2 marks
   because he is complaining of a clear discharge from his nose. The
   discharge tests positive for beta-2 transferrin. What is the problem
   and what should be done about it?
e. The patient is also noted to have swelling and pain in his right ear. The   2 marks
   emergency department doctor thinks this is a pinna haematoma. How
   should this be managed and what is the outcome if it is not treated?

10) A 47-year-old female with a history of recurrent ear infections is referred to the ENT clinic because her primary care doctor is concerned about a cholesteatoma.

a.	Define cholesteatoma.	1 mark
b.	Describe how a cholesteatoma invades.	2 marks
c.	Give two signs the doctor might see on otoscopy.	2 marks
d.	State two investigations that should be carried out.	2 marks
e.	Name three possible complications of a cholesteatoma.	3 marks

11) An 8-year-old male is seen by his primary care doctor with a midline lump in his neck. He is normally very well and has not had any trauma to his neck. The doctor diagnoses a thyroglossal cyst.

a.	Describe how a thyroglossal cyst is formed.	3 marks
b.	Give two features of a thyroglossal cyst on examination.	2 marks
c.	State one imaging method used to confirm the diagnosis.	1 mark
d.	Name three other causes of midline neck lumps.	3 marks
e.	State one method to treat this condition.	1 mark

12) A 5-year-old boy is sent to the emergency department from his primary care doctor because he has a high temperature and looks unwell. When he is assessed by the paediatrician, a diagnosis of mastoiditis is suspected.

a.	What are two signs the paediatrician may find on examination?	2 marks
b.	What is the underlying pathological process?	2 marks
c.	Name two investigations that would be helpful in this case.	2 marks
d.	State three methods to manage acute mastoiditis.	3 marks
e.	Name one complication that may result after treatment.	1 mark

13) A 29-year-old veterinary nurse presents to her primary care doctor with midfacial pain which has been present for 3 days. She also has a congested nose, sore throat and cough. On examination, her observations are normal and there are no other abnormalities. The doctor diagnoses acute rhinosinusitis.

a. What is the most likely aetiology?   1 mars
b. State three methods to manage this patient.   3 marks
c. The patient returns a week later and complains that she is feeling   1 mark
   worse. She has developed a red, swollen left eye and says her vision
   is blurred. On examination, there is restriction of eye movements.
   What complication has developed?
d. Name three more complications of acute sinusitis.   3 marks
e. State two further management strategies for this patient.   2 marks

Chapter 8

Trauma and orthopaedics
QUESTIONS

Single best answer questions

1) What percentage of total body calcium is stored within bone?

a.   1%.
b.   25%.
c.   75%.
d.   99%.

2) The patella is an example of which type of bone?

a.   Long bone.
b.   Short bone.
c.   Sesamoid bone.
d.   Flat bone.

3) A 23-year-old male attends the emergency department with a 1-hour history of pain in his left foot. He is struggling to weight-bear. A Simmonds' test shows no movement on squeezing the left calf. What is the most likely diagnosis?

a. Lisfranc injury.
b. Pes cavus.
c. Plantar fasciitis.
d. Achilles tendon rupture.

4) A 56-year-old male attends the emergency department with a 5-hour history of pain in the buttock, posterior thigh and calf. On examination, he has a restricted straight leg raise. Bowels and urinary systems are intact. What is the most likely diagnosis?

a. Cauda equina.
b. Disc prolapse.
c. Bacterial discitis.
d. Spinal stenosis.

5) A 42-year-old male presents to his primary care doctor with a reduced ability to turn his head. On examination, he has prominent winging of the scapula. Which nerve has been affected to cause this appearance?

a. Axillary nerve.
b. Suprascapular nerve.
c. Long thoracic nerve.
d. Anterior interosseous nerve.

6) A 42-year-old attends his primary care doctor with a 1-week history of back pain. He underwent a knee arthroscopy 5 days ago under a spinal anaesthetic. On examination, he is pyrexial at 38.2°C and he is tender on his back at the level of L1/L2. What is the most likely diagnosis?

a. Bacterial discitis.
b. Scoliosis.
c. Spinal tuberculosis.
d. Prolapsed intervertebral disc.

7) Which classification system is used to describe paediatric fractures that involve the growth plate?

a. Weber.
b. Salter-Harris.
c. Garden.
d. Schatzker.

8) Which knee compartment is most commonly affected in osteoarthritis?

a. Medial compartment.
b. Lateral compartment.
c. Anterior compartment.
d. Tibial compartment.

9) A 62-year-old male attends the orthopaedic clinic with a vague history of back pain and weakness in his legs. Pain is worse on standing or walking on a slope. Symptoms have increased over the past 2 months. What is the most likely diagnosis?

a.   Spondylolisthesis.
b.   Disc prolapse.
c.   Spinal stenosis.
d.   Cauda equina.

10) A 32-year-old female attends the clinic with a 5-week history of shoulder pain and difficulty holding objects in her hand. On examination, she has wasting of the intrinsic muscles of her hand and paraesthesia in the medial side of the arm. What is the most likely diagnosis?

a.   Carpal tunnel syndrome.
b.   Apical lung cancer.
c.   Rheumatoid arthritis.
d.   Osteoarthritis.

11) If the deep peroneal nerve is damaged, what sign may be observed?

a.   Trendelenburg gait.
b.   Loss of proprioception distally.
c.   Lack of sensation on the sole of the foot.
d.   Foot drop.

12) Fractures of which part of the scaphoid are at highest risk of avascular necrosis?

a. Proximal pole.
b. Waist.
c. Distal pole.
d. Posterior segment.

13) According to the British Orthopaedic Association Standards for Trauma, a patient admitted with an open tibial fracture should have the defect covered with which of the following dressings?

a. Cling film.
b. Sterile drape.
c. Saline-soaked gauze.
d. The wound should not be covered.

14) A 56-year-old male attends his primary care doctor with a 2-week history of pain in his elbow. He is a keen sports player. On examination, he has tenderness over the medial epicondyle of the humerus. What is the most likely diagnosis?

a. Olecranon bursitis.
b. Cubitus valgus.
c. Tennis elbow.
d. Golfer's elbow.

15) A 25-year-old male is referred from his primary care doctor with a 2-month history of back pain radiating to the buttocks with progressive back stiffness. On examination, he has a reduced range of all spinal movements. Blood tests show a raised ESR and CRP. Spinal X-ray notes sacroiliac sclerosis and new intervertebral syndesmophytes. What is the most likely diagnosis?

a. Ankylosing spondylitis.
b. Disc prolapse.
c. Rheumatoid arthritis.
d. Scoliosis.

16) What is the most common type of shoulder dislocation?

a. Posterior dislocation.
b. Anterior dislocation.
c. Inferior dislocation.
d. Superior dislocation.

17) A 32-year-old male attends the emergency department following a fall onto an outstretched hand. On examination, he has pain in the anatomical snuffbox and on wrist movements. What is the most likely diagnosis?

a. Ganglion.
b. Perilunate dislocation.
c. Scaphoid fracture.
d. Colles' fracture.

18) The Weber classification is used to aid in the management of ankle fractures. What is a Weber B fracture?

a. A stable injury.
b. An unstable injury.
c. A fracture without damage to the soft tissues.
d. Either stable or unstable, depending on the associated soft tissue injury.

19) Which of the following does not form part of the rotator cuff?

a. Supraspinatus.
b. Teres major.
c. Infraspinatus.
d. Subscapularis.

20) A 62-year-old female with osteoarthritis presents to her primary care doctor with a swelling behind her knee. On examination, she has a fluctuant mass posterior to the midline at the level of the joint; this mass is tense on extension and soft on flexion. What is the underlying diagnosis?

a. Popliteal aneurysm.
b. Infrapatellar bursitis.
c. Prepatellar bursitis.
d. Popliteal cyst.

21) Which structure travels through the carpal tunnel?

a. Radial artery.
b. Abductor pollicis brevis.
c. Flexor carpi ulnaris.
d. Flexor pollicis longus.

22) Which of the following is NOT supplied by the ulnar nerve?

a. Interosseous muscles.
b. Flexor digitorum profundus to the ring finger.
c. Opponens pollicis.
d. Medial two lumbricals.

23) A 56-year-old male is admitted with an intracapsular neck of femur fracture. With no other information, what is the least likely surgical treatment to be offered?

a. Cannulated screw fixation.
b. Long intramedullary nail.
c. Total hip arthroplasty.
d. Hemiarthroplasty.

Extended matching questions

Paediatric orthopaedic conditions

a. Osgood-Schlatter's disease.
b. Osteochondritis dissecans.
c. Ewing's sarcoma.
d. Osteomyelitis.

e. Achondroplasia.
f. Juvenile idiopathic arthritis.
g. Transient tenosynovitis.
h. Septic arthritis.

Match the description of the patient with the most likely diagnosis.

1) A 13-year-old boy with hip pain, particularly at night. He has a raised WCC and is anaemic. X-rays show a lytic lesion with a periosteal reaction in the proximal femur with a characteristic onion skin appearance.

2) A 3-year-old presents with a new-onset limp and left hip pain. She has been suffering with a viral illness for the last 5 days. Her bloods show a mild inflammatory reaction but she cries when you externally rotate her hip. USS shows a small effusion.

3) A 4-year-old child has been unable to weight-bear on his left leg for the last 24 hours. His knee is too painful to examine and he is febrile with a raised WCC and CRP. He was completely well up until 24 hours ago.

4) A 12-year-old physically active boy presents with an 18-month history of knee pain. MRI shows small cracks in the articular cartilage and subchondral bone shows early signs of avascular necrosis.

5) A 14-year-old long-distance runner presents with anterior knee pain which is worse when running and gets better with rest. He has a prominent tibial tuberosity and pain over the patella ligament.

Knee injuries

a.   ACL rupture.   e.   Bipartite patella.
b.   PCL rupture.   f.   Patella fracture.
c.   Medial meniscus tear.   g.   Osteoarthritis.
d.   Quadriceps tendon rupture.   h.   Tibial plateau fracture.

Match the presentation of the patient with the most likely diagnosis.

6)   A 28-year-old rugby player twisted his knee 3 days ago when he planted his foot and turned quickly to avoid a tackle. He heard a popping sound and his knee swelled up almost immediately. He now complains of instability.

7)   A 63-year-old male, who was walking down a steep hill, lost his footing and fell forwards onto a flexed knee. The following morning it was swollen and very sore to walk on. He can bend his knee but can't lift his foot up off the couch. You aspirate a couple of millilitres of straw-coloured fluid from his knee.

8)   A 55-year-old male, who was cycling downhill, came off his bike and fell forwards onto a flexed knee. That evening, it was swollen and very sore to walk on. He can't bend his knee or lift his leg up off the couch without pain. You aspirate 30ml blood from his knee which has fat globules on the surface. There is no obvious fracture on plain X-ray.

9)   A 72-year-old female slips in the supermarket on a wet floor, landing on a flexed knee. There is some bruising and swelling; despite this, she is weight-bearing with difficulty but can't lift her foot off the examination couch. She has point tenderness over the patella, but nowhere else.

10) A 27-year-old male complains of his right knee locking for the last 3 months following a football tackle in which his primary care doctor said he had a medial collateral ligament injury. He is not able to run anymore without pain but is still able to go about his daily life. On examination, he is sore around the medial joint line and his knee clicks. He has no instability on a valgus stress test and is yet to have any imaging of his knee.

Hip pain

a.	Pathological fracture.	e.	Appendicitis.
b.	Osteoarthritis.	f.	Rheumatoid arthritis.
c.	Perthes' disease.	g.	Septic arthritis.
d.	Slipped upper femoral epiphysis.	h.	Psoas abscess.

Match the description of the patient with the most likely diagnosis.

11) A mother brings her 7-year-old non-verbal autistic son to you from the primary care doctor. For the last 24 hours, he has been walking hunched over, has vomited twice with a low-grade fever and is in considerable pain when you move his right hip. He has not eaten today and normally has a good appetite. He was in no pain prior to this and he will not let you examine his abdomen.

12) A 72-year-old male with known Paget's disease presents with 4 weeks of progressive pain in his right hip. He was walking with difficulty until yesterday when he fell to the floor and couldn't get up.

13) A 5-year-old boy presents to you in clinic with a new limp for the last 3 weeks. He has reduced and painful internal rotation of the hip. He is otherwise fit and well and his X-rays are unremarkable.

14) A 38-year-old intravenous drug user has felt non-specifically unwell for the last 3 days. He has a temperature of 38.3°C, a WCC of 23 x 10^9/L and CRP of 250mg/L. He can't flex his right hip due to pain.

15) An 18-month-old toddler is brought in with a 3-day history of limping. She is now non-weight-bearing and has a low-grade fever. Her WCC and CRP are elevated. Her hip is incredibly painful to move and feels warm.

Chest pain in trauma patients

a. Rib fractures.   e. Psychosomatic chest pain.
b. Myocardial infarction.   f. Gastric ulcer.
c. Pulmonary embolism.   g. Fat embolism syndrome.
d. Sternal fracture.   h. Pericarditis.

Match the description of the patient with the most likely diagnosis.

16) A 22-year-old male came off his bike whilst overtaking a car, hitting the right side of his chest on the kerb. His chest wall is bruised and incredibly painful to touch. His saturations are normal and his chest X-ray is normal.

17) A 54-year-old smoker fell out of the loft a week ago. He broke a couple of ribs and has been taking regular naproxen which is the only thing helping the pain. He has been experiencing retrosternal chest pain for the last 2 days, which he has put down to referred pain from the rib fractures. He wants some stronger pain relief.

18) A 34-year-old motorcyclist has sustained an open multifragmented tibia and fibula fracture in a road traffic collision at high speed. At the roadside, the paramedics had to put a tourniquet on to stem the blood loss from a likely arterial injury. Three days postoperatively, he develops low saturations, confusion and a petechial rash across his chest.

19) A 31-year-old patient with a history of anxiety is admitted with an anterior shoulder dislocation following a fall from height. You have just explained that you would like to attempt to reduce her dislocation in the department using Entonox®. While you are getting the equipment ready, she develops widespread chest pain and tachypnoea. The ECG is normal and the ABG shows a respiratory alkalosis.

20) An 89-year-old patient presents with a 1-hour history of sudden-onset chest pain. She underwent a cemented hemiarthroplasty earlier today. The operation took longer than usual and blood loss was >500ml. The anaesthetist commented that she was struggling to maintain the patient's cardiac output intra-operatively.

Treatment of neck of femur fractures

a. Cemented hemiarthroplasty.
b. Uncemented hemiarthroplasty.
c. Cannulated screws.
d. Long intramedullary nail.
e. Short intramedullary nail.
f. Dynamic hip screw (DHS).
g. Total hip replacement.
h. Non-surgical treatment.

Match the description with the most appropriate treatment option.

21) A 72-year-old female who walks about a mile per day with her dogs has a displaced intracapsular neck of femur fracture. She had some moderate osteoarthritis on the X-ray and she says she gets good days and bad days with her hip.

22) A 55-year-old male who still cycles to work, fell from his bike and sustained a valgus impacted intracapsular neck of femur fracture.

23) A 68-year-old female with breast cancer sustains an intertrochanteric neck of femur fracture through an area of abnormal bone. A full-length femur view shows a lytic lesion further down the shaft.

24) An 82-year-old male who walks with a Zimmer frame sustains a simple two-part intertrochanteric fracture. The bone is osteopenic but structurally normal.

25) A 79-year-old bed-bound female with severe dementia and aortic stenosis fell whilst being hoisted. She has sustained a displaced intracapsular neck of femur fracture. The family don't want her to have an operation because she's "suffered enough".

Splints, casts and braces

a.   Above-knee backslab.   e.   Thumb spica.

b.   Below-knee backslab.   f.   Futura splint.

c.   Above-elbow backslab.   g.   Richard's splint (extension).

d.   Below-elbow dorsal backslab.   h.   Range of movement knee brace.

Match the description of the patient with the most likely diagnosis.

26) An 85-year-old female with a Colles' type fracture of the distal radius. A cast is likely to be her definitive treatment.

27) A 28-year-old skier with a Bennett's type fracture.

28) A 13-year-old with a spiral distal tibia fracture.

29) A 48-year-old male with a likely quadriceps tendon rupture.

30) A 59-year-old with bilateral wrist fractures. Her left wrist (non-dominant) is being treated non-operatively in a below-elbow plaster of Paris (POP) cast. Her right wrist is going to be plated later on today.

Upper limb injuries

a.	Acute rotator cuff tear.	e.	Proximal humerus fracture.
b.	Degenerative rotator cuff tear.	f.	Anterior dislocation.
c.	Frozen shoulder.	g.	Long head of biceps rupture.
d.	Labral tear.	h.	Calcific tendonitis.

Match the description of the patient with the most likely diagnosis.

31) A 92-year-old female fell over in her kitchen. The whole upper arm is bruised with a clear anterior joint line swelling. She is able to externally rotate and abduct her arm but it is painful. X-rays are awaited.

32) A 63-year-old retired mechanic with an 8-month history of shoulder pain. He has a full range of movement but has weakness of internal and external rotation against resistance. He denies any previous trauma.

33) A 43-year-old hairdresser with 6 months of difficulty lifting her arms above her head. She has normal strength in all muscle groups but finds initiating abduction painful. Her X-ray shows an opacity in the subacromial space.

34) A 19-year-old who is a spin bowler for the county cricket team, has had 3 months of shoulder pain whilst bowling. He has normal strength but he has some anterior instability. His X-rays are normal.

35) A 39-year-old epileptic patient has shoulder pain following a seizure this morning. There is a fullness in the anterior joint line, squaring of the affected shoulder and she is unable to externally rotate her arm.

Elbow pathologies

a.	Tennis elbow.	e.	Osteoarthritis.
b.	Golfer's elbow.	f.	Distal biceps tendon rupture.
c.	Olecranon bursitis.	g.	Median nerve compression.
d.	Ulnar nerve compression.	h.	Gout.

Match the description of the patient with the most likely diagnosis.

36) A 57-year-old dinner lady with 6 months of elbow pain. She has point tenderness over the origins of extensors carpi radialis longus and brevis. She has had to go onto light duties at work and it is not getting any better.

37) A 27-year-old carpenter who was lifting a box at work and felt a sudden pop in his elbow. His arm was very bruised and swollen and he is now having trouble at work particularly with using a screwdriver.

38) A 62-year-old male who can no longer straighten his elbow. He gets intermittent pain in the joint usually at night. He remembers having an elbow fracture as a young man which was treated in plaster.

39) A 3-year-old child with a supracondylar fracture which she sustained on holiday in France 2 weeks ago and she has been in an above-elbow plaster cast since. Her hand is warm and pink but not sweaty like the other hand. She is unable to make the 'OK' sign.

40) A 21-year-old with a painless swelling over the back of the elbow which he noticed during exam season at university. It is not red, nor painful.

Chapter 8 | Trauma and orthopaedics EMQs

Brachial plexus and nerve injuries

a. Erb's palsy.
b. Klumpke's palsy.
c. Lateral cord injury.
d. Radial nerve palsy.

e. Ulnar nerve palsy.
f. Inferior root palsy.
g. Median nerve neuropraxia.
h. Posterior cord compression.

Match the description of the patient with the most likely diagnosis.

41) A cyclist came off his motorbike 2 months ago, was dragged a short distance and broke his cervical spine in several places. He is still unable to hold a pen and has notice wasting of the small muscles of his hand. You noticed a Horner's syndrome.

42) During a routine CT aortic angiogram prior to vascular surgery, the radiologist noted an aneurysm in the second part of the axillary artery. The patient has weakness of shoulder abduction and wrist extension.

43) Three months after a stab injury in the antecubital fossa, the patient still has numbness over the thenar eminence and struggles to hold heavy shopping bags.

44) A 56-year-old female developed weakness of wrist extension 2 weeks following an open reduction, internal fixation of a humeral fracture. She was able to extend her wrist pre-operatively. She is still able to straighten her fingers.

45) A 2-week-old baby born by forceps delivery does not appear to be moving his right arm.

Short answer questions

1) A 41-year-old secretary is referred by her primary care doctor with tingling in her thumb and index finger in the middle of the night. She is struggling to hold heavy shopping bags and feels like she is often having to stop typing at work to shake her hands until the feeling comes back. She feels tired all the time and it is really starting to get her down.

a. What is carpal tunnel syndrome and with respect to the relevant anatomy, explain her symptoms?   3 marks

b. Name two groups at risk of developing carpal tunnel syndrome.   2 marks

c. Give three treatment options for this patient.   3 marks

d. Name two risks of carpal tunnel decompression surgery.   1 mark

e. State one investigation that may be relevant in this case.   1 mark

2) A 4-year-old child is brought to the emergency department by her teacher who is worried that her elbow is very swollen, bruised and deformed. The child said she fell off a climbing frame 4 days ago and it has been painful ever since. She said she had told her father and her grandmother but they did not think it was anything serious.

a. How many joints form the elbow joint and name these?   4 marks

b. What is the most likely injury for this patient?   1 mark

c. What nerve is most at risk in this injury and why?   1 mark

d. Having appropriately managed her injury in the emergency department, would you admit this child? Please state your reasoning.   2 marks

e. Due to a delayed presentation, she developed a malunion. State two limitations she would experience.   2 marks

3) A 52-year-old retired rugby player is referred to orthopaedic outpatients with osteoarthritis of his right knee.

a. State two X-ray findings for osteoarthritis. 2 marks

b. The majority of disease is localised to the medial compartment. What 1 mark surgical procedure is appropriate?

c. Specify two ways an implant may degenerate over time. 2 marks

d. He presents to the emergency department 4 weeks after surgery with 3 marks a red, hot, swollen knee. His wound is well healed but he feels unwell and has been spiking fevers. Name three immediate management options.

e. He returns to your clinic 15 years later. It is clear his implant has worn 2 marks out. State two treatment options.

4) A 30-year-old male fell from scaffolding whilst intoxicated 24 hours ago. He is admitted with a Weber C ankle fracture. He is in a below-knee backslab and has his leg elevated on a pillow. He keeps leaving the ward for a cigarette and coming back with pain.

a. State one effect smoking has on bone healing. 1 mark

b. Name two implications of operating if the ankle is too swollen. 2 marks

c. After 5 days of elevation, the ankle is still too swollen to operate. 2 marks State two management options.

d. Postoperatively, the patient complains of excruciating pain and the 3 marks nurses are concerned. State three ways to assess the patient.

e. You suspect compartment syndrome. State the appropriate 2 marks treatment for this patient.

5) A 3-year-old boy is admitted to the emergency department with a 48-hour history of a painful right hip and he is crawling rather than walking. He has been well up until 2 days ago. His mother says he has been very warm, but still shivering. He was born prematurely at 32 weeks but otherwise has no health conditions. His bloods show a CRP of 350mg/L and his temperature is 38.9°C.

a. Give three potential causes of new-onset limping in children. 2 marks

b. Describe the epidemiology of Perthes' disease. 1 mark

c. State two X-ray findings for Perthes' disease. 2 marks

d. Name three other investigations to establish the diagnosis. 3 marks

e. Name the most common causative organism in paediatric 2 marks osteomyelitis and what is the treatment.

6) An 86-year-old female is brought to the emergency department following a fall whilst shopping. She has a dinnerfork deformity of her wrist, which is swollen, painful and starting to bruise.

a. What injury is being described and state two associated radiological 3 marks findings?

b. Give two areas in a neurovascular assessment. 2 marks

c. Describe how you would reduce this fracture. 3 marks

d. Name two specific risks of open reduction and internal fixation of the 1 mark wrist.

e. State one factor to influence your decision to admit or discharge the 1 mark patient.

7) A 46-year-old medical secretary attends her primary care doctor with a 4-week history of swollen and painful hands which is now interfering with her work. The doctor suspects she has osteoarthritis.

a. Give two examples of osteoarthritic changes in the hands. 2 marks

b. Give two examples of hand changes in rheumatoid arthritis. 2 marks

c. State two examples of surgical and two examples of non-surgical 4 marks
treatments for osteoarthritis of the hands.

d. Describe the deformity of mallet finger. 1 mark

e. What is Dupytren's contracture? 1 mark

8) A 19-year-old male born in Nigeria, but who has lived in the UK for the last 10 years, presents with a 3-week history of thoracic back pain and fevers.

a. Define Pott's disease. 1 mark

b. Name two X-ray features which may suggest TB of the spine. 2 marks

c. Describe how TB may spread from the lungs to the vertebral bodies 3 marks
and the process which leads to vertebral body collapse.

d. State two ways in which sickle cell disease can affect bone. 2 marks

e. Name two sexually transmitted diseases affecting the skeleton. 2 marks

9) A 29-year-old male who competes in the national judo team is seen in the fracture clinic 3 days after he had had a shoulder dislocation reduced. During the match, his opponent picked him up and threw him to the floor landing on top of him.

a. Name two anatomical structures that act to keep the humeral head in 2 marks
the glenohumeral joint.

b. What type of dislocation is he most likely to have sustained and how 2 marks
would you confirm this?

c. State three initial treatments for this patient. 3 marks

d. What are the chances of him redislocating? 1 marks

e. Name one functional consequence of recurrent dislocation and one 2 marks
X-ray finding suggestive of recurrent dislocation.

10) A 73-year-old female is admitted to the emergency department following a fall whilst walking her dog in the snow. She landed on her left hip. An X-ray is performed which shows a moderately displaced intracapsular neck of femur fracture.

a.   Describe the bony anatomy of the hip with respect to the trochanters 2 marks
     and capsular attachments.

b.   Describe the blood supply to the hip, starting from the external iliac 3 marks
     arteries. Why is this important when considering displaced
     intracapsular neck of femur fractures?

c.   State one treatment option and what one factor that might influence 2 marks
     your decision.

d.   Given how fit she is, with no past medical history, a non-smoker, an 2 marks
     active badminton player who already has moderately severe arthritis,
     what treatment should she be offered and why?

e.   What weight-bearing status would you recommend for each 1 mark
     treatment option for this type of injury?

11) A 26-year-old male is admitted to the emergency department following a road traffic accident in which he came off his motorbike at 70mph falling onto both hands. On examination, both forearms are deformed, his left hand is cold, pale and has a large defect on the radial border of his forearm. The right wrist is swollen and deformed.

a.   State two immediate management options for the left hand.   2 marks

b.   What is a Galeazzi type fracture?   1 mark

c.   His right wrist shows a displaced, comminuted intra-articular distal 3 marks
     radius fracture. You can see the emergency department consultant
     measuring various heights and angles around the wrist joint. State the
     normal values for radial height, inclination and volar tilt.

d.   Which of the injuries carry the worst prognosis and why?   2 marks

e.   The patient would like to return to his own county which is a 2-hour   2 marks
     drive away. What kind of immobilisation would you prescribe for each
     fracture?

12) A 23-year-old male attends the emergency department
    following a bar fight. He has a large laceration in his left
    antecubital fossa. He is drunk and combative in the
    department and it is difficult to assess.

a.   State three structures that are at risk within the antecubital fossa in   3 marks
     penetrating trauma.

b.   The patient is unable to flex his wrist against resistance. What injury   2 marks
     has occurred and where is this located?

c.   If the ulnar nerve is damaged within the forearm, what functional   2 marks
     deficit within the hand can he expect?

d.   He comes back to the clinic 3 months after the injury and is having   2 marks
     real difficulty in lifting heavy objects and his bicep muscle bulk
     appears quite proximal. What could he have injured and how would
     you investigate this?

e.   What functional deficit may he continue to complain of longer term,   1 mark
     despite repair of the above injury?

13) A 43-year-old female is referred to the spinal clinic by her
    primary care doctor following the diagnosis of an L5 nerve
    root compression.

a.   Define the terms 'radiculopathy' and 'myelopathy'.   2 marks

b.   State two examination findings you may find in this patient.   1 mark

c.   What nerve roots are being tested in the biceps, triceps, knee and   4 marks
     ankle reflexes?

d.   Where would you test lower limb dermatomes L3 and L4?   2 marks

e.   State the nerve that supplies the muscles responsible for ankle   1 mark
     dorsiflexion.

Chapter 9

Fluids and electrolytes
QUESTIONS

Single best answer questions

1) The interstitial and plasma fluid form which compartment?

a. Intracellular.
b. Extracellular.
c. Third space.
d. Peripheral space.

2) For a typical 70kg male what is the total body water content?

a. 18L.
b. 28L.
c. 35L.
d. 42L.

3) What is the normal daily requirement for water and electrolytes?

a. 3.0L water, 150mmol sodium, 30mmol potassium in 24 hours.
b. 3.0L water, 100mmol sodium, 60mmol potassium in 24 hours.
c. 2.5L water, 100mmol sodium, 60mmol potassium in 24 hours.
d. 2.5L water, 150mmol sodium, 30mmol potassium in 24 hours.

4) What is the volume of the intracellular fluid compartment?

a. 3.5L.
b. 15.5L.
c. 23L.
d. 28L.

5) What is the most abundant extracellular cation?

a. Sodium.
b. Potassium.
c. Calcium.
d. Magnesium.

6) What is the most abundant intracellular cation?

a. Sodium.
b. Potassium.
c. Phosphate.
d. Calcium.

7) An 80-year-old male attends the emergency department following review of his recent blood results by his primary care doctor. He takes amiloride for hypertension. Which of the following electrolyte abnormalities would his doctor be concerned about?

a. Hypokalaemia.
b. Hyperkalaemia.
c. Hyponatraemia.
d. Hypernatraemia.

8) A 42-year-old female is admitted to the emergency department with a 4-day history of diarrhoea and vomiting. She has had very little to eat for the past 4 days and her ECG notes a broad T wave with the presence of U waves in several leads. What is the underlying electrolyte disorder?

a. Hypokalaemia.
b. Hyperkalaemia.
c. Hyponatraemia.
d. Hypernatraemia.

9) A 25-year-old male is admitted to the endocrine ward with hypotension, hypoglycaemia and vomiting. His bloods show a sodium level of 123mmol/L and a potassium level of 6.7mmol/L. What is the underlying cause of his electrolyte disturbance?

a. Secondary hyperaldosteronism.
b. Cushing's syndrome.
c. Addison's disease.
d. Primary hyperaldosteronism (Conn's syndrome).

10) With regards to the potassium level in question 9, what is the most important action to perform first to protect the myocardium?

a. Calcium resonium.
b. 10ml 10% calcium gluconate.
c. Insulin and dextrose infusion.
d. Salbutamol nebuliser.

11) With regards to the potassium level in question 9, which of these treatments will be most effective at driving potassium into cells?

a. Calcium resonium.
b. 10ml 10% calcium gluconate.
c. Insulin and dextrose infusion.
d. Salbutamol inhaler.

12) A 2-week-old baby experiences projectile vomiting after each feed and shows signs of poor growth and development. The vomiting is non-bilious in nature. On examination, an olive-shaped mass is felt in the right upper abdominal quadrant. An ultrasound shows a target sign confirming the diagnosis of pyloric stenosis. What electrolyte disturbances are commonly associated with this condition?

a. Hypokalaemic metabolic alkalosis.
b. Hyperkalaemic metabolic acidosis.
c. Hypokalaemic hypochloraemic metabolic alkalosis.
d. Hypernatraemic hypochloraemic metabolic acidosis.

13) A 53-year-old male has been admitted to the surgical ward following an elective right hemicolectomy on the same day. The doctor on-call has reviewed his bloods which show: Hb 110g/L (previously 135g/L), sodium 132mmol/L, potassium 3.0mmol/L, creatinine 70μmol/L and urea 4.3mmol/L. He has vomited twice since surgery. What would be the most appropriate management option?

a.   40mmol IV potassium chloride in 0.9% sodium chloride over 8 hours.
b.   40mmol IV potassium chloride in Hartmann's solution over 8 hours.
c.   40mmol IV potassium chloride in 0.9% sodium chloride over 3 hours.
d.   No management required.

14) You are a junior doctor on the urology ward. The nurses contact you as a 60-year-old male has returned from theatre 2 hours ago and appears to be confused, restless and vomiting. On further questioning, the nurses reveal he has undergone a transurethral resection of the prostate which was a complex procedure lasting for 1.5 hours. You contact your senior colleague who suspects TURP syndrome. What electrolyte abnormality is found in this condition?

a.   Hypernatraemia.
b.   Hyperkalaemia.
c.   Hypocalcaemia.
d.   Hyponatraemia.

15) A 35-year-old female is admitted to the ward with persistent vomiting and diarrhoea. The ward medical team has prescribed four 1L bags of 5% dextrose to be given over 8 hours for each bag. Two days later, bloods are taken and it is noted that she has a sodium of 125mmol/L which has fallen from 135. What would be the most appropriate management option in this patient?

a. Slow IV 0.9% sodium chloride.
b. Slow IV 18% sodium chloride.
c. Fluid restriction.
d. Repeat bloods the following day.

16) Prior to performing the action in question 15, the medical doctor on-call asks for blood tests looking at serum osmolality, urinary osmolality and urinary sodium. What would you expect to find on these results if the hyponatraemia was due to excessive fluid therapy?

a. Decreased serum osmolality, decreased urinary osmolality and decreased urinary sodium.
b. Decreased serum osmolality, increased urinary osmolality and increased urinary sodium.
c. Decreased serum osmolality, normal urinary osmolality and normal urinary sodium.
d. Increased serum osmolality, increased urinary osmolality and increased urinary sodium.

17) Which of the following would cause a positive Trousseau sign?

a. Hypercalcaemia.
b. Hypocalcaemia.
c. Hyperphosphataemia.
d. Hyperkalaemia.

18) Which of the following ECG changes is seen in hypocalcaemia?

a. Prolonged QT interval.
b. Absent P waves.
c. Presence of U waves.
d. Tall tented T waves.

19) Which of the following is not a cause of hyperphosphataemia?

a. Chronic renal failure.
b. Tumour lysis syndrome.
c. Myeloma.
d. Refeeding syndrome.

20) Which of the following is not a symptom of hypercalcaemia?

a. Abdominal pain.
b. Chvostek's sign.
c. Depression.
d. Renal stone formation.

21) A 72-year-old male being treated for a metastatic bronchial carcinoma is admitted to the emergency department with increased vomiting, abdominal pain and generalised weakness. An ECG shows a shortened QT interval. His blood results show a raised calcium level at 2.68mmol/L. Which of the following would not be a suitable management option?

a. IV 0.9% sodium chloride.
b. IV bisphosphonates.
c. IV calcium gluconate.
d. Haemodialysis.

22) A 23-year-old male is brought into resus following a road accident. He has a compound fracture to his right tibia and multiple lacerations. During the A-E assessment, his blood pressure is noted to be 80/40mmHg and gradually declining. The consultant in charge asks a junior doctor to prescribe an appropriate resuscitation fluid. Which of the following would be the most appropriate and has the correct fluid classification?

a. Crystalloid — type-specific blood.
b. Colloid — sodium chloride.
c. Colloid — albumin.
d. Crystalloid — Hartmann's solution.

23) A 64-year-old male is admitted to the medical ward following a collapse at home. He notes some abdominal pain and multiple episodes of vomiting at home. An abdominal X-ray confirms the findings of a small bowel obstruction. The patient informs the team he has not opened his bowels for 7 days and has eaten little in this time. An NG tube is inserted and parenteral nutrition is commenced. Two days later he has deranged liver function tests, erratic blood sugars and a fall in serum sodium, potassium, magnesium and phosphate. What is the diagnosis?

a. Normal response to reintroduction of feed.
b. Acute cholecystitis.
c. Refeeding syndrome.
d. Bowel perforation.

Extended matching questions

Daily fluid requirements

a.	200ml.	e.	15ml/kg.
b.	350ml.	f.	25ml/kg.
c.	1500ml.	g.	100mmol.
d.	2000ml.	h.	140mmol.

Match the volume with the appropriate requirement or loss.

1) Normal daily urinary volume.

2) Normal daily water loss in faeces.

3) Insensible water losses by the respiratory tract.

4) Normal daily requirement of sodium.

5) Daily maintenance fluid requirement per kg of body weight per day.

Fluid composition

a.   5mmol/L.   e.   154mmol/L.
b.   76mmol/L.   f.   5g.
c.   124mmol/L.   g.   50g.
d.   131mmol/L.   h.   500g.

Match the correct electrolyte concentration to each 1L of solution.

6)   Sodium content in Hartmann's solution.

7)   Sodium content in 0.9% sodium chloride (normal saline).

8)   Potassium content in Hartmann's solution.

9)   Chloride content in 0.9% sodium chloride (normal saline).

10) Grams of dextrose in 5% dextrose.

Cellular ions

a.	Sodium.	e.	140mmol.
b.	Potassium.	f.	150mmol.
c.	Magnesium.	g.	0.0000001mmol.
d.	Calcium.	h.	120mmol.

Match the correct cellular ion/concentration to the description below.

11) What is the most abundant intracellular cation?

12) Which cellular ion has a total body level of 4200mmol?

13) What is the intracellular potassium concentration?

14) What is the extracellular sodium concentration?

15) What is the intracellular calcium concentration?

Appropriate use of fluids

a.	Sodium bicarbonate.	e.	Hartmann's solution.
b.	0.9% sodium chloride/5% glucose.	f.	Albumin.
c.	5% dextrose.	g.	Blood.
d.	0.9% sodium chloride.	h.	Gelofusin®.

Match the most appropriate fluid option to each description.

16) A crystalloid fluid containing 5mmol of potassium.

17) This fluid is often used as a maintenance fluid in neonates.

18) This fluid is prepared by hydrolysis of bovine collagen.

19) If used in excess can cause a hyperchloraemic metabolic acidosis.

20) This colloid has a strict transfusion protocol and bloods must be taken before use.

Signs of electrolyte disturbances

a.	Hypokalaemia.	e.	Hypocalcaemia.
b.	Hyperkalaemia.	f.	Hypercalcaemia.
c.	Hyponatraemia.	g.	Hypophosphataemia.
d.	Hypernatraemia.	h.	Hyperchloraemia.

Match the appropriate sign with the electrolyte disturbance.

21)   Chvostek and Trousseau's signs.

22)   Prolonged QT interval.

23)   Tall tented T waves.

24)   U waves.

25)   Prolonged PR interval.

Managing electrolyte imbalances

a. 20% human albumin.
b. Calcium resonium.
c. 10% calcium gluconate.
d. 0.9% sodium chloride.

e. Sando-phos.
f. Sando-K®.
g. Hypertonic saline.
h. Blood.

Match the appropriate option for each electrolyte imbalance.

26) Drug used to stabilise the myocardium in hyperkalaemia.

27) Rehydration therapy used in hypercalcaemia.

28) Used in the treatment of severe hyponatraemia with features such as seizures.

29) Oral alternative in the treatment of hypokalaemia.

30) A treatment for a patient with hypovolaemic hypernatraemia.

Drugs and electrolyte imbalance

a.	Hypokalaemia.	e.	Hypocalcaemia.
b.	Hyperkalaemia.	f.	Hypercalcaemia.
c.	Iron overload.	g.	Hypophosphataemia.
d.	Hypoglycaemia.	h.	Hypervitaminosis D.

Match the appropriate electrolyte to the drug or drug class given.

31) Loop diuretics such as furosemide can lead to this electrolyte imbalance.

32) ACE inhibitors such as ramipril can lead to this electrolyte imbalance.

33) Amiloride and spironolactone can lead to this electrolyte imbalance.

34) Thiazide diuretics such as bendroflumethiazide can cause this electrolyte imbalance.

35) Acute digoxin toxicity can lead to this electrolyte imbalance.

Causes of electrolyte imbalances

a. Refeeding syndrome.
b. IV contrast.
c. Renal failure.
d. Milk-alkali syndrome.

e. Oral iodine.
f. Conn's syndrome.
g. Appropriate use of IV fluids.
h. Vitamin B_{12} deficiency.

Match the most likely cause of each electrolyte disorder below.

36) Hyperkalaemia.

37) Hypernatraemia.

38) Hyperphosphataemia.

39) Hypercalcaemia.

40) Hypophosphataemia.

Acid base disorders

a. Renal tubular acidosis.   e. Head injury.
b. Normal tidal breathing.   f. Diabetic ketoacidosis.
c. Vomiting.   g. Mild alcohol ingestion.
d. Hyperventilation.   h. Mild cellulitis.

Match the diagnosis with the most likely cause.

41) Metabolic acidosis with a high anion gap.

42) Metabolic alkalosis.

43) Respiratory acidosis.

44) Respiratory alkalosis.

45) Metabolic acidosis with a low anion gap.

Short answer questions

1) A 25-year-old male is brought into the emergency department following a road traffic accident. His airway is patent and his lungs are clear with good air entry bilaterally. His blood pressure is 80/40mmHg with a pulse of 120 bpm. His capillary refill time is 4 seconds and he appears pale. The doctor suspects the patient is in hypovolaemic shock.

a. Name one crystalloid fluid which may be used for resuscitation.   1 mark
b. If the above fluid fails to produce a sustained rise in blood pressure,   1 mark
    what other fluid treatment could be considered?
c. The patient is stabilised and transferred to the ward for further   3 marks
    management. The junior doctor on-call is asked to prescribe him daily
    maintenance fluids as he has been vomiting. Specify three questions
    to consider prior to prescribing any fluids.
d. Name three routes of daily water loss.   3 marks
e. List the concentrations of sodium, chloride, potassium, lactate,   2 marks
    calcium, glucose and osmolarity of 0.9% sodium chloride and
    Hartmann's solution.

2) A 72-year-old male is recovering from a transurethral resection of the prostate (TURP). He has had little fluid intake since the procedure and nursing staff are concerned and ask a doctor to prescribe fluids. He is prescribed 4 bags of 1L 0.9% sodium chloride over 16 hours. The following day he becomes short of breath and has ankle swelling. His catheter is draining well, blood pressure is stable and saturations are 93% on room air; blood tests show no abnormalities. A diagnosis of iatrogenic fluid overload is made.

a. Name three things you would expect to find on examination in   3 marks
    pulmonary oedema.
b. Which investigation could the doctor order to confirm the diagnosis?   1 mark
c. Name two treatments other than diuretics that could be used to   2 marks
    relieve symptoms.
d. Identify two common complications of loop diuretics.   2 marks
e. Explain the pathophysiology behind TURP syndrome.   2 marks

3) A 45-year-old female is seen in the emergency department after presenting to her primary care doctor with a 1-week history of diarrhoea and vomiting; she appeared drowsy in clinic. Bloods taken show a sodium of 130mmol/L. The blood test was repeated as the doctor was unsure if it was taken from the same arm as an active IV fluid line; the repeat sample shows a sodium of 128mmol/L.

a. Give six other causes of hyponatraemia.   3 marks
b. Name two other symptoms of hyponatraemia.   2 marks
c. Name two investigations for hyponatraemia.   2 marks
d. Give two treatments of hypervolaemic hyponatraemia.   2 marks
e. Name one complication due to rapid changes in sodium levels.   1 mark

4) A 48-year-old male presents to his primary care doctor with weight gain, bruising to his skin, recurrent infections, tiredness, abdominal striae and weakness in his extremities. He undergoes a range of tests including electrolytes, 24-hour urinary cortisol and a dexamethasone suppression test which confirms the diagnosis of Cushing's syndrome.

a. Name two electrolyte abnormalities in Cushing's syndrome.   2 marks
b. What is the difference between Cushing's disease and Cushing's   1 mark
    syndrome?
c. Specify three symptoms and three signs of hypernatraemia.   3 marks
d. Give one treatment for hypovolaemic hypernatraemia.   1 mark
e. Name three complications of hypernatraemia.   3 marks

5) A 45-year-old male is admitted to the emergency department with diarrhoea and vomiting. He has had very little to eat or drink over the past 3 days. He is clinically dehydrated and you request bloods including electrolytes. His blood results show: potassium 3.1mmol/L, sodium 134mmol/L, urea 8.1mmol/L, creatinine 140μmol/L.

a. Please interpret the above blood results.   2 marks
b. Name four other causes of hypokalaemia.   2 marks
c. Name two symptoms and two signs of hypokalaemia.   2 marks
d. Suggest two findings which may be present on an ECG.   2 marks
e. Give two treatment options for an asymptomatic patient.   2 marks

6) A 21-year-old female attends the emergency department following a collapse. The paramedics noted she appeared drowsy since they arrived and she complained of abdominal pain at home. Observations show a blood pressure of 90/60mmHg, with a pulse of 110 bpm. On examination, muscle wasting and areas of hyperpigmentation are evident. The doctor requests several blood tests and the results show: potassium 5.8mmol/L, sodium 121mmol/L, urea 4.1mmol/L, creatinine 70μmol/L. An ABG is performed which shows a metabolic acidosis.

a. Interpret the above results and state an appropriate diagnosis.   2 marks
b. Name four causes of hyperkalaemia.   2 marks
c. What three findings may be present on an ECG?   3 marks
d. Which drug is given to stabilise the myocardium?   1 mark
e. Name two treatments used to lower potassium levels.   2 marks

7) An 82-year-old male is admitted to the emergency department with increased confusion, increasing thirst for the past 3 days and signs of dehydration. He is currently under treatment for a metastatic lung cancer. His blood results show a calcium of 2.65mmol/L, and a raised phosphate and alkaline phosphatase.

a. Interpret the above results and state an appropriate diagnosis.   2 marks
b. Name one sign and one symptom of mild, moderate and severe hypercalcaemia.   3 marks
c. What two treatments may be used to reduce his calcium level?   2 marks
d. Suggest one cause of primary hyperparathyroidism.   1 mark
e. What are the changes in PTH and serum calcium in the above condition?   2 marks

8) A 40-year-old male has recently undergone a total thyroidectomy. He returns to the clinic 3 weeks later and his bloods show a calcium level of 2.11mmol/L and a low PTH.

a.	Interpret the above results and state an appropriate diagnosis.	2 marks
b.	Name three signs that may be seen in hypocalcaemia patients.	3 marks
c.	Which electrolyte should be corrected concurrently if low?	1 mark
d.	Specify two changes seen on the ECG in this patient.	2 marks
e.	Provide two causes of a high PTH and low calcium.	2 marks

9) A 35-year-old female was admitted with persistent vomiting for 48 hours. An ABG was taken to assess for acid-base status whilst on room air.

	Result	Normal values
pH	7.59	7.35-7.45
PaCO$_2$	5.1	4.7-6.0kPa
HCO$_3^-$	36	24-30mmol/L
PaO$_2$	12	11-13 on room air
Base excess	+4	+/- 2mmol/L
Anion gap	13	12-16mmol/L

a.	Please interpret the above ABG.	2 marks
b.	Name three causes of this acid-base disturbance.	3 marks
c.	Specify two possible signs of this acid-base disorder.	2 marks
d.	Name one complication of this acid-base disorder.	1 mark
e.	What methods of compensation would return the pH to a normal range?	2 marks

10) A 19-year-old male was admitted to the emergency department following a 1-day history of polydipsia, polyuria, abdominal pain and vomiting. He is assessed and the junior doctor requests the following ABG taken on room air.

	Result	Normal values
pH	7.27	7.35-7.45
$PaCO_2$	4.82	4.7-6.0kPa
HCO_3^-	16	24-30mmol/L
PaO_2	13	11-13 on room air
Base excess	-5	+/- 2mmol/L
Anion gap	18	12-16mmol/L

a. Please interpret the above ABG.   2 marks
b. Name two causes of this acid-base disturbance.   1 mark
c. Specify two symptoms and one sign of this acid-base disorder.   3 marks
d. How would you calculate the anion gap?   1 mark
e. Name three causes of a normal anion gap and three causes of a raised   3 marks
    anion gap.

11) A 68-year-old female with COPD presents to the emergency department with shortness of breath. She has an ABG performed which shows the following result.

	Result	Normal values
pH	7.31	7.35-7.45
$PaCO_2$	6.9	4.7-6.0kPa
HCO_3^-	26	24-30mmol/L
PaO_2	8.4	11-13 on room air
Base excess	-1	+/- 2mmol/L
Anion gap	14	12-16mmol/L

a.   Please interpret the above ABG.   3 marks
b.   Name two causes of this acid-base disturbance.   2 marks
c.   Name one symptom of this acid-base disorder.   1 mark
d.   Name two complications of this acid-base disorder.   2 marks
e.   How would you differentiate between a Type I and Type II respiratory   2 marks
     failure?

12) A 72-year-old male is admitted with shortness of breath.
     An ABG is taken to assess for admission to hospital and
     provide baseline observations.

	Result	Normal values
pH	7.43	7.35-7.45
PaCO$_2$	6.2	4.7-6.0kPa
HCO$_3^-$	22	24-30mmol/L
PaO$_2$	14	11-13 on room air
Base excess	0	+/- 2mmol/L
Anion gap	14	12-16mmol/L

a.   Please interpret the above ABG.   2 marks
b.   Name three causes of this acid-base disturbance.   3 marks
c.   Specify one symptom and one sign of this acid-base disorder.   2 marks
d.   Name one complication of this acid-base disorder.   1 mark
e.   What methods of compensation would return the pH to a normal   2 marks
     range?

13) A 66-year-old male is admitted to the emergency department with shortness of breath, fever and a productive cough for 48 hours. He has noted some confusion. His respiratory rate is 18 and his urea is 8.1mmol/L. A chest X-ray notes consolidation in the right lower zone consistent with pneumonia. His CURB-65 score is 3. Three days into his admission he informs staff he feels excessively thirsty and has not been passing as much urine as usual and it appears dark. Clinically he does not appear dehydrated. The medical consultant is concerned about syndrome of inappropriate ADH secondary to pneumonia.

a.   Name four other causes of this condition.   4 marks

b.   Describe the underlying pathology in this condition.   2 marks

c.   Specify what would be seen on a urine sample.   2 marks

d.   What class of drugs is usually used to treat this condition?   1 mark

e.   Which condition is associated with rapid correction of electrolyte   1 mark
     abnormalities?

Section 2
Answers

Chapter 10

Upper GI surgery
ANSWERS

Single best answers

1)   a.
2)   a.
3)   c.
4)   d.
5)   b.
6)   a.
7)   b.
8)   c.
9)   a.
10)   b.
11)   b.
12)   c.
13)   a.
14)   c.
15)   a.
16)   c.
17)   b.
18)   b.
19)   b.
20)   d.

21) a.
22) c.
23) b.

Extended matching question answers

1) d

   Severe vomiting leads to a tear in the mucosa at the junction of the stomach and the oesophagus. It is usually a self-limiting condition but may require surgical or endoscopic treatment.

2) b

   The history of epigastric pain relieved by eating indicates that the patient has a peptic ulcer. These are divided into duodenal ulcers which are relieved with food and gastric ulcers which are worsened with food. Treatment involves prescribing proton pump inhibitors or H2 receptor antagonists and addressing the underlying cause such as *H. pylori*, NSAIDs and smoking. Endoscopic intervention is required in bleeding ulcers.

3) a

   A history of an upper GI bleed combined with a history of alcohol excess and signs of chronic liver failure should indicate oesophageal varices as the cause of this patient's bleeding.

4) e

   This patient has an aorto-enteric fistula which is a communication between a repaired aorta and GI tract. It should be considered in any patient who has a history of an open or endovascular repair of an aortic aneurysm. It can result in bloody stools and even death.

5) h

   This is an uncommon cause for an upper GI bleed; however, pernicious anaemia is a risk factor for gastric adenocarcinoma. The enlarged hard left supraclavicular lymph node is Troisier's sign indicating a metastatic abdominal malignancy.

6)   a
Acute pancreatitis is the inflammation of the pancreas. It is commonly caused by gallstones and alcohol. The mnemonic 'I GET SMASHED' can be used to remember the causes of pancreatitis. Symptoms include epigastric pain radiating to the back which is severe in nature and exacerbated by eating, fever or jaundice. Treatment is supportive with fluids, analgesia and maintaining nutrition; nasojejunal feeding is used.

7)   c
Biliary colic is pain occurring when the gallbladder contracts against an obstruction which is usually a stone in Hartmann's pouch. The pain occurs following ingestion of fatty foods and may be associated with nausea and vomiting. Patients are usually otherwise well and blood tests are unremarkable.

8)   e
These are congenital bile duct abnormalities due to cystic dilation of the biliary tree. They are often diagnosed at birth but approximately 20% of cases are diagnosed in adults. They are classified based on the site and are treated by cyst removal. If left untreated, they may lead to pancreatitis or recurrent cholangitis.

9)   f
Charcot's triad of jaundice, fever and right upper quadrant pain are the key features of ascending cholangitis. The addition of confusion and hypotension to the other factors of Charcot's triad is known as Reynolds' pentad.

10) g

A liver abscess is the collection of pus within the liver parenchyma as a result of bacterial, fungal or parasitic infection. The history of swinging pyrexia should make you suspicious of an abscess. *Entamoeba histolytica* is associated with an amoebic liver abscess. Treatment involves antibiotics and aspiration.

11) h

Patients with Peutz-Jeghers syndrome develop multiple hamartomatous polyps in the gastrointestinal tract. They often have mucocutaneous pigmentation. The polyps are prone to malignant transformation.

12) f

A carcinoid is a neuroendocrine tumour affecting the gastrointestinal system which produces serotonin (5-HT). It is common at the appendix or terminal ileum but may occur at any point along the GI tract. Symptoms include abdominal pain, GI bleeding, flushing, hypotension and weight loss. Patients can be treated with somatostatin analogues such as octreotide.

13) d

Small bowel lymphomas are most commonly found in the ileum. Primary lymphomas are resected whilst secondary small bowel lymphomas are treated with chemotherapy.

14) a

Adenomas are associated with familial adenomatous polyposis which is a condition associated with a mutation in the APC tumour suppressor gene. Patients have multiple bowel adenomas, and frequently develop colorectal cancer at an early age. These patients require frequent screening.

15) b

Gastrointestinal stromal tumours are rare accounting for less than 1% of all primary GI tumours. They are associated with a mutation in the C-KIT gene and can be managed with a combination of resection, chemotherapy, radiofrequency ablation and imatinib therapy.

16) h

This history of previous acute cholecystitis and swinging pyrexia indicates that this patient has a gallbladder empyema. An empyema is the presence of pus within a cavity. A gallbladder empyema usually occurs due to a stone becoming lodged within the gallbladder outlet during an episode of acute cholecystitis. This condition is a surgical emergency and requires urgent drainage.

17) e

Acute cholecystitis results from gallstones obstructing bile flow out of the gallbladder; this results in inflammation. Typical symptoms include right upper quadrant pain, fever, a raised WCC and a positive Murphy's sign. The treatment involves antibiotics and removal of the gallbladder which should be performed on hospital admission, within 2 weeks of presentation or delayed for at least 6 weeks to allow time for the inflammation to resolve prior to performing the procedure.

18) d

This patient has a gallstone obstructing the common bile duct and the most appropriate treatment is to remove the stone using endoscopic retrograde cholangiopancreatography (ERCP).

19) g

Laparoscopic cholecystectomy is the gold standard of treatment for acute cholecystitis. Current guidelines advocate this procedure to be performed during the same hospital admission or within 2 weeks of diagnosis.

20)   d

Charcot's triad of jaundice, fever and right upper quadrant pain are the key features of ascending cholangitis. It is an infection of the biliary tree and commonly occurs due to obstruction. Treatment is with antibiotics and removal of the obstruction using ERCP.

21)   d

A complication of pancreatitis is the formation of a pseudoaneurysm due to damage in local blood vessels by pancreatic enzymes which can lead to haemorrhage. Treatment involves radiological embolisation.

22)   a

Adult respiratory distress syndrome (ARDS) is a syndrome of non-cardiogenic pulmonary oedema and lung inflammation. A chest X-ray will show bilateral opacifications and patients will require admission to critical care for ventilatory support. It is essential to monitor fluid balance, urine output and central venous pressure.

23)   h

Exocrine pancreatic insufficiency is the inability to digest food due to a lack of pancreatic digestive enzymes. It is often found in conditions such as cystic fibrosis and chronic pancreatitis.

24)   b

A pseudocyst is a collection of amylase-rich fluid enclosed within fibrous or granulation tissue. Patients may present with epigastric pain or a palpable mass. Pseudocysts may resolve spontaneously but may require surgical drainage if they do not resolve.

25)   g

The radiological findings suggest an infection within non-viable pancreatic tissue. Pancreatitis can lead to necrosis and if this is infected it usually leads to sepsis and multi-organ failure.

26) d

A highly selective vagotomy aims to remove only the vagal stimulation to the parietal cell mass in the body of the stomach to reduce acid secretion but preserve gastric emptying.

27) a

A Billroth I procedure involves the removal of the pylorus, and the distal stomach is anastomosed directly to the duodenum which results in better protein and fat digestion compared to a Billroth II procedure; however, this results in a higher level of gastric outlet obstruction.

28) f

A Roux-en-Y procedure is commonly used in weight loss surgery. The creation of a small stomach pouch ensures that large amounts of food cannot be consumed and bypassing the duodenum means that fat absorption is greatly reduced.

29) c

This procedure involves eliminating the vagal stimulation to the stomach which reduces acid secretion but leads to gastric paralysis which requires a further procedure such as a pyloroplasty or gastrojejunostomy to be performed to ensure adequate stomach drainage.

30) b

A Billroth II procedure involves the anastomosis of the greater curvature of the stomach to the first part of the jejunum following resection of the lower end of the stomach. It is indicated in refractory peptic ulcer disease and gastric adenocarcinoma.

31) e

Adenocarcinoma and squamous cell carcinoma are the most common forms of oesophageal malignancy. The progressive history of dysphagia to solids and then liquids indicates an increasing obstruction to the oesophagus and combined with weight loss should point towards malignancy. Adenocarcinoma usually occurs in the lower third of the oesophagus and is associated with smoking, alcohol consumption, obesity, Barrett's oesophagus, gastro-oesophageal reflux disease and nitrosamine ingestion.

32) b

The history of an acutely unwell patient with the radiology findings indicate an oesophageal perforation.

33) a

The bird's beak appearance on barium swallow is characteristic for achalasia which is an oesophageal motility disorder in which there is a failure of lower oesophageal sphincter relaxation and there is a loss of oesophageal peristalsis.

34) f

Adenocarcinoma and squamous cell carcinoma are the most common forms of oesophageal malignancy. The progressive history of dysphagia to solids and then liquids indicates an increasing obstruction to the oesophagus and combined with weight loss should point towards malignancy. Squamous cell carcinoma usually occurs in the upper two thirds of the oesophagus and is associated with smoking, alcohol, achalasia, coeliac disease and Plummer-Vinson syndrome.

35) c

A peptic stricture is a complication of longstanding gastro-oesophageal reflux disease. Chronic irritation of the oesophageal mucosa leads to fibrosis and stricture. Management includes endoscopic balloon dilatation, antacids and in recurrent cases surgical resection.

36) a
A carcinoid is a neuroendocrine tumour affecting the gastrointestinal system which produces serotonin (5-HT). It is common at the appendix or terminal ileum but may occur at any point along the GI tract. Symptoms include abdominal pain, GI bleeding, flushing, hypotension and weight loss. Patients can be treated with somatostatin analogues such as octreotide.

37) g
Adenocarcinoma and squamous cell carcinoma are the most common forms of oesophageal malignancy. The progressive history of dysphagia to solids and then liquids indicates an increasing obstruction to the oesophagus and combined with weight loss should point towards malignancy. Squamous cell carcinoma usually occurs in the upper two thirds of the oesophagus and is associated with smoking, alcohol, achalasia, coeliac disease and Plummer-Vinson syndrome.

38) c
Gastrointestinal stromal tumours are rare accounting for less than 1% of all primary GI tumours. They are associated with a mutation in the c-KIT gene and can be managed with a combination of resection, chemotherapy, radiofrequency ablation and imatinib therapy.

39) b
Patients with Peutz-Jeghers syndrome develop multiple hamartomatous polyps in the gastrointestinal tract. They often have mucocutaneous pigmentation. The polyps are prone to malignant transformation.

40) f

Adenocarcinoma and squamous cell carcinoma are the most common forms of oesophageal malignancy. The progressive history of dysphagia to solids and then liquids indicates an increasing obstruction to the oesophagus and combined with weight loss should point towards malignancy. Adenocarcinoma usually occurs in the lower third of the oesophagus and is associated with smoking, alcohol consumption, obesity, Barrett's oesophagus, gastro-oesophageal reflux disease and nitrosamine ingestion.

41) g

Platelet counts peak at 7-10 days following a splenectomy. Aspirin may be indicated for very high platelet counts above 1000g/dL.

42) c

The history of a swinging pyrexia, mild overlying erythema and progressive splenomegaly indicates a splenic abscess. The history of bacterial endocarditis is a risk factor as bacteraemia is the most common predisposing factor. A splenectomy is the treatment of choice for these patients.

43) a

Howell-Jolly and Pappenheimer bodies are an indication of hyposplenism. Pappenheimer bodies are abnormal basophilic granules of iron found inside red blood cells, whilst Howell-Jolly bodies are the presence of basophilic nuclear remnants in circulating erythrocytes.

44) f

A laparoscopic approach is increasingly used for an elective splenectomy as there is a decrease in postoperative complication rates, reduced postoperative pain, a shortened recovery time and decreased hospital stay.

45) b

This patient demonstrates features of hypersplenism. It is usually treated initially with medical management; however, if this fails then a splenectomy is indicated.

Short answer question answers

1)

a. Fever. 3 marks

Right upper quadrant pain.

Jaundice.

b. Cholangitis is inflammation, normally due to infection, of an 1 mark
obstructed bile duct.

c. Any 2 from: 1 mark

- Gallstones.
- Head of pancreas malignancy.
- Primary sclerosing cholangitis.
- Cholangiocarcinoma.
- Bile duct stricture.

d. Any 3 from: 3 marks

- AKI.
- Sepsis.
- Encephalopathy.
- Coagulopathy.
- Hepatic failure.
- Renal failure.
- Malabsorption.

e. Gram-negative sepsis (1 mark). When the biliary tree is obstructed, 2 marks
intraluminal pressure can rise to >20mmHg causing small gaps to
open up between the cells lining the vessel allowing bacteria in. There
are other theories including bile backing up into the liver meaning
Kupffer cells (specialised macrophages in the liver) cannot work
efficiently leading to SIRS (1 mark).

2)

a. The majority of gallstones are mixed but can be made of cholesterol   2 marks
    and bile pigments.

b. Bilirubin is a byproduct of haem metabolism, from the breakdown of   3 marks
    red blood cells (1 mark). It travels bound to albumin to the liver where
    it is conjugated to glucuronic acid (1 mark). Now soluble, it is excreted
    through bile into the bowel where it is further metabolised to
    urobilinogen and stercobilinogen (1 mark). Both are responsible for
    pigmenting urine and stools, respectively.

c. Ultrasound is the usual first-line investigation.   1 mark

d. The patient could undergo an ERCP to remove the stone but the risk   3 marks
    of precipitating pancreatitis in a young person can be as high as 20%.
    In an appropriate centre, the preferred option might be an on-table
    cholangiogram (OTC) and laparoscopic CBD exploration.

e. Any 2 from: 1 mark

    ● Acute pancreatitis.
    ● Cholecystitis.
    ● Cholangitis.

3)

a. Any 3 from: 3 marks

    ● Remain upright after meals.
    ● Avoid fatty/spicy foods.
    ● Stop smoking.
    ● Lose weight.
    ● Leave at least 4 hours between an evening meal and bed.
    ● Diary of symptoms and foods that may trigger it.

b. Barrett's oesophagus affects the lower third of the oesophagus and is   2 marks
    characterised by metaplasia of the stratified squamous epithelium to
    simple columnar epithelium.

c. Adenocarcinoma.   2 marks
    Squamous cell carcinoma.

d. Alcohol.   2 marks
    Smoking.
e. Endoscopic stenting to allow food to pass and relieve symptoms.   1 mark

4)

a. Acute pancreatitis.   1 mark
b. Any 3 from: 3 marks
    - Analgesia.
    - IV fluids.
    - Oxygen.
    - Catheterisation
c. Any 1 from: 1 mark
    - Modified Glasgow Score.
    - Ranson Score.
    - APACHE II.
    - Balthazar.
d. Any 3 from: 3 marks
    - Sliding scale insulin.
    - Artificial nutrition.
    - Antibiotics.
    - ERCP.
    - Ventilatory support.
    - Haemofiltration.
    - Inotropic support.
e. Acute 2 from: 2 marks
    - Pancreatic necrosis.
    - Sepsis.
    - Pancreatic pseudocyst.
    - Acute respiratory distress syndrome (ARDS).
    - Disseminated intravascular coagulation (DIC).
    - Renal failure.
    - Haemorrhage.
    - Pseudoaneurysm.
    - Malnutrition.

- Systemic inflammatory response syndrome (SIRS).
- Multi-organ failure.
- Diabetes mellitus.
- Exocrine pancreatic insufficiency.
- Chronic pancreatitis.
- Hyperglycaemia.
- Hypocalcaemia.
- Shock.

5)

a. Any 3 from: 3 marks

- Trauma.
- Spontaneous rupture.
- Hypersplenism.
- Hydatid cysts.
- Splenic abscess.
- Neoplasia.

b. Any 2 from: 2 marks

- Antibiotic prophylaxis.
- Immunisation.
- Aspirin.
- Advice regarding seeking urgent medical advice at the early signs of infection.

c. Any 3 from: 3 marks

- *Streptococcus pneumoniae.*
- *Haemophilus influenzae.*
- *Neisseria meningitidis.*
- *Salmonella typhi.*
- *Escherichia coli.*
- *Klebsiella pneumoniae.*
- *Streptococcus agalactiae.*

d. Overwhelming post-splenectomy infection. 1 mark

e. A splenunculus is a small nodule of splenic tissue that is separate from 1 mark the rest of the organ; they are found in approximately 10% of the population.

6)

a. Any 4 from: 2 marks

- *Helicobacter pylori.*
- Ischaemia.
- Burns.
- Stress.
- Prolonged critical care stay.
- Zollinger-Ellison syndrome.
- Long-term NSAID use.
- Steroids.
- Smoking.
- Excess alcohol.
- Chronic gastritis.

b. Any 3 rows from Table 10.1.   3 marks

Table 10.1

	Gastric ulcer	Duodenal ulcer
Male:female ratio	3:1	5:1
Presentation age	50 years	25-30 years
Relationship to food	Pain on eating food	Pain relieved by food
Vomiting	Pain relieved by vomiting	Rare
Cyclical	Not cyclical	Can occur in cycles which last approximately 2 weeks
Abdominal pain	Epigastric	Epigastric

c. Gastroscopy.   1 mark

d. Any 1 from: 1 mark
    - Haemorrhage.
    - Perforation.
    - Stricture.
    - Malignant change.
    - Obstruction.

e. Any 3 from: 3 marks
    - Stop smoking.
    - Reduce alcohol intake.
    - Avoid NSAIDs.
    - *H. pylori* eradication therapy.
    - Antacids.
    - Proton pump inhibitors (PPI).
    - H2 antagonists.
    - Surgery.

7)

a. Gastric cancer.   1 mark

b. Troisier's sign is an enlarged hard left supraclavicular lymph node   1 mark
    which indicates a metastatic abdominal malignancy.

c. Any 4 from: 4 marks
    - *H. pylori* infection.
    - Blood group A.
    - Diet low in vitamin C.
    - Hypogammaglobulinaemia.
    - Intestinal metaplasia.
    - Gastric polyps.
    - Gastric dysplasia.
    - Pernicious anaemia.
    - Previous gastric resection.
    - Previous gastric ulceration.
    - Atrophic gastritis.

d.   TNM staging assesses the size of the tumour, the presence of lymph   3 marks
     nodes and the evidence of metastases.

e.   Any 1 from: 1 mark
     - CT scan.
     - Ultrasound.
     - Endoscopic ultrasound.
     - Laparoscopy.

8)

a.   Any 2 from: 2 marks
     - Epigastric pain.
     - Weight loss.
     - Steatorrhoea.
     - Diabetes mellitus.

b.   Any 2 from: 2 marks
     - Serum amylase.
     - Abdominal X-ray.
     - CT.
     - MRCP.
     - ERCP.

c.   Any 1 from: 1 mark
     - Pancreatic enlargement.
     - Fibrosis.
     - Calcification.

d.   Any 4 from: 4 marks
     - Low-fat diet.
     - Avoid alcohol.
     - Analgesia.
     - Pancreatic enzyme supplementation.
     - Insulin therapy.
     - Fat-soluble vitamins.

e.   Pain team.   1 mark

9)

a. Any 2 from: 1 mark
- Increased age.
- Obesity.
- Pregnancy.
- Ascites.
- Coughing.
- Increased diaphragmatic hiatus.
- Loss of diaphragmatic tone.

b. Sliding. 2 marks
Rolling.

c. Sliding: dyspepsia and vomiting. 4 marks
Rolling: dyspepsia, odynophagia, dyspnoea on eating, dyspnoea on bending down.

d. Any 2 from: 2 marks
- Proton pump inhibitor.
- Weight loss.
- Alteration in diet.
- Smoking cessation.
- Reduce alcohol intake.
- Fundoplication.

e. Any 2 from: 1 mark
- Incarceration.
- Strangulation.
- Gastric volvulus.

10)

a. Small bowel obstruction. 1 mark

b. Any 3 from: 3 marks
- Hernia.
- Adhesions.
- Malignancy.
- Volvulus.

- Congenital bands.
- Gallstone ileus.
- Food bolus.
- Parasites.
- Intussusception.
- Bezoar.
- Congenital atresia.
- Crohn's disease.

c. Any 2 from: 2 marks
- IV fluids.
- NG tube.
- Catheterisation.

d. Urgent laparotomy.   2 marks

e. Any 2 from: 2 marks
- Dehydration.
- Electrolyte disturbances.
- AF.
- Bowel necrosis.
- Bowel perforation.
- Peritonitis.
- Death.

11)

a. Hepatocellular carcinoma.   1 mark

b. α-fetoprotein (AFP).   1 mark

c. Any 4 from: 4 marks
- Hepatitis B.
- Hepatitis C.
- Viral hepatitis.
- Cirrhosis.
- Mycotoxins (aflatoxin) cirrhosis.
- Liver adenoma.
- Haemochromatosis.

- Anabolic steroids.
- Oral contraceptives.
- Primary sclerosing cholangitis.
- α1-antitrypsin deficiency.

d. Any 2 from: 2 marks
- Serum AFP.
- CT.
- Ultrasound liver.
- MRI.
- Liver biopsy.

e. Any 2 from: 2 marks
- Surgical resection.
- Transplant.
- Chemoembolisation.
- Systemic chemotherapy.

12)

a. Any 4 from: 4 marks
- Biliary stricture.
- Biliary atresia.
- Gallstones.
- Pancreatitis.
- Cholangiocarcinoma.
- Primary sclerosing cholangitis.
- Carcinoma of the head of the pancreas.

b. Carcinoma of the head of the pancreas (2 marks).   2 marks
Pancreatic cancer (1 mark).

c. Multidisciplinary team (MDT) discussion.   1 mark

d. Pancreaticoduodenectomy.   2 marks
Whipple's procedure.

e. Any 1 from: 1 mark
- Palliative ERCP with stenting.
- Percutaneous transhepatic cholangiogram with stenting.

- Surgical bypass.
- Palliative care team review.
- Palliative chemotherapy.

13)

a.   Gastro-oesophageal reflux disease.   1 mark

b.   Any 4 from: 4 marks

- Obesity.
- Smoking.
- Alcohol.
- Stress.
- Family history.
- Hiatus hernia.
- Gastroparesis.
- High caffeine intake.
- Pregnancy.
- Calcium channel blockers.
- Oestrogen usage.
- Gastroparesis.
- Beta-adrenergic agonists.
- Previous gastric surgery.
- Nitrites.

c.   Any 2 from: 2 marks

- Symptoms worse on bending.
- Pain after alcohol consumption.
- Pain after hot liquid ingestion.
- Regurgitation.
- Pain after a large meal.
- Sore throat.
- Chronic cough.
- Halitosis.
- Hoarse voice.

d. Any 2 from: 2 marks
- PPI trial.
- Upper GI endoscopy.
- Barium study.
- Oesophageal pH monitoring.
- Oesophageal manometry.
- Gastric emptying studies.

e. Any 1 from: 1 mark
- Barrett's oesophagus.
- Adenocarcinoma.
- Oesophageal stricture.
- Pulmonary fibrosis.
- Chronic cough.
- Asthma.
- Chronic pain.

Chapter 11

Lower GI surgery
ANSWERS

Single best answers

1) b.
2) c.
3) c.
4) b.
5) d.
6) d.
7) d.
8) b.
9) b.
10) b.
11) a.
12) c.
13) b.
14) d.
15) b.
16) b.
17) c.
18) b.
19) c.
20) b.

21) d.
22) c.
23) a.

Extended matching question answers

1) g

This is faecal loading.

2) h

This is a sign of bowel inflammation.

3) a

This sign is caused by a large loop of dilated sigmoid colon which has the appearance of a coffee bean.

4) e

This sign is where both sides of the bowel wall can be visualised on X-ray as there is air on both sides due to a pneumoperitoneum caused by a perforated viscus.

5) b

Valvulae conniventes can be seen across the full diameter of small intestine, while haustra only reach across part of the diameter of large intestine.

6) b

The anaemia and altered blood in the stool suggest this patient is losing blood from a right-sided tumour.

7) h

These symptoms in a young patient suggest IBD.

8)   d

Being overweight is a risk factor for haemorrhoids.

9)   a

The pain associated with fresh bleeding suggests a fissure.

10)   f

This patient's bleeding is fresh red, suggesting it is left-sided. The weight loss would cause concern that it is a tumour rather than diverticular disease.

11)   d

Ileus is common after abdominal surgery.

12)   f

Sigmoid volvulus is more common in patients with learning disabilities. It causes symptoms and signs of obstruction.

13)   b

These symptoms fit with gastroenteritis. *Campylobacter* is a common cause of gastroenteritis.

14)   c

This patient will be on opiate analgesia which is a common cause of constipation.

15)   e

These symptoms should cause concern for a malignancy as there is a recent change in bowel habit; the change from constipation to watery diarrhoea suggests a tumour is partially obstructing the bowel and overflow diarrhoea has occurred.

16) d

This patient's age and symptoms fit with diverticulitis. The pneumoperitoneum suggests a perforated diverticulum.

17) e

This patient has pain and fever and has recently returned from the operating theatre, so there should be a suspicion of a retained foreign body.

18) a

In this case, the possibilities are ovarian cyst rupture and appendicitis, but the latter is more likely with the right-sided guarding, vomiting and loss of appetite.

19) b

This patient has signs of faecal loading.

20) f

Gastroenteritis may cause abdominal pain and in the absence of other symptoms this is the most likely diagnosis.

21) c

Grey-Turner's sign may indicate a retroperitoneal haemorrhage.

22) f

Rebound tenderness indicates peritonitis.

23) e

The psoas sign indicates irritation of the iliopsoas group of hip flexor muscles signifying a retrocaecal appendicitis.

24) d

Murphy's sign has a high sensitivity for cholecystitis. It is usually negative in pyelonephritis, ascending cholangitis and choledocholithiasis.

25) g

Rigler's sign is seen on an abdominal radiograph indicating air on the luminal and peritoneal side of the bowel wall. It indicates a pneumoperitoneum due to perforation, surgery or instrumentation.

26) e

This patient's weight gain is most likely simple obesity. As she has not had a period for 4 years, she is unlikely to be pregnant.

27) g

In a man of this age, these symptoms and signs may be caused by a ruptured abdominal aortic aneurysm. This is an emergency so should not be missed.

28) b

Radiotherapy can lead to complications such as a stricture in the bowel. In this case, this occurred due to the proximity of the area being treated (prostate) to the rectum and has resulted in obstruction.

29) h

The blood in the stools and the mass suggest a malignancy. This case is complicated with a shortness of breath and chest pain which as such may indicate a pulmonary embolism.

30) a

A shifting dullness suggests the distention is caused by fluid, e.g. ascites. Ulcerative colitis is associated with primary sclerosing cholangitis, so this may be causing liver failure resulting in ascites.

31) b

Most patients with a prolapse initially only notice it after opening their bowels and it retracts in between. Faecal incontinence is a common symptom. COPD is a risk factor as patients will cough frequently, putting more strain on the pelvic floor muscles.

32) f

Pilonidal sinuses develop in hair follicles in the natal cleft. They are more common in men, particularly with more hair growth in the area. If they become infected, a pilonidal abscess develops.

33) c

The discharge this patient is experiencing is coming from the cutaneous end of a fistula in ano, which connects the anus to the skin. They are more common in patients with diverticular disease.

34) a

Children can develop anal fissures. They are very painful and can cause bleeding.

35) e

This is a perianal abscess as it is not in the right location for a pilonidal abscess. This patient is predisposed to developing an abscess due to his obesity and diabetes.

36) c

Lynch syndrome is also known as hereditary non-polyposis colon cancer (HNPCC). It is associated most strongly with colorectal cancer and endometrial cancer, as well as ovarian, pancreatic, skin, prostate and bladder tumours. Inheritance is autosomal dominant so the gene has been inherited from the mother and the father is unaffected.

37) g

Peutz-Jeghers syndrome causes multiple hamartomas in the small intestine and typical buccal and perioral pigmentation. There is an increased risk of colorectal and small intestinal cancer. Inheritance is autosomal dominant.

38) b

Familial adenomatous polyposis leads to the development of hundreds of polyps throughout the colon. There is a 100% risk of progression to cancer if untreated, so patients are offered a prophylactic total colectomy at a young age.

39) a

Cowden disease results in hamartomas on the skin and mucous membranes, and an increased risk of some cancers including breast and thyroid. Most patients have gastrointestinal polyps or other abnormalities.

40) d

Li-Fraumeni syndrome gives an increased risk of developing sarcomas, leukaemia, brain tumours, breast cancer and tumours of the adrenal cortex. There is also an increased risk of some other cancers including colorectal. This family tree fits the diagnostic criteria for Li-Fraumeni syndrome.

41) a

This patient will not be a candidate for surgery due to his advanced cancer. Palliative management would be most appropriate.

42) g

This patient has a right-sided colonic tumour. A right hemicolectomy is the best operation to remove this with good excision margins.

43)   h

This patient has inflammation throughout his colon and has developed a bowel perforation as a complication of his ulcerative colitis. In this situation, medical management will not treat the problem sufficiently and a total colectomy is needed to remove the diseased bowel.

44)   b

This patient has a low rectal tumour which can be palpated on examination so an anterior resection is appropriate. This operation removes the rectum and a temporary stoma may be formed or the sigmoid colon may be anastomosed to the stump.

45)   a

This patient has gastroenteritis so only symptomatic management is required.

Short answer question answers

1)

a. Diverticulosis is the presence of diverticulae in the bowel wall. 1 mark
Diverticulitis is inflammation of diverticulae.

b. CT of the abdomen. 1 mark

c. Any 4 from: 4 marks
- Initially she should only have clear fluids to rest the bowel and allow the inflammation to settle.
- IV fluids should be given.
- Diet can then be gradually reintroduced when symptoms improve.
- IV antibiotics should be given to cover intra-abdominal infection, according to local guidelines.
- Analgesia should be given to control pain.
- If any complications develop, surgery would be needed but otherwise she could be managed conservatively.
- Following discharge she should have a flexible sigmoidoscopy after 6-8 weeks to exclude any other cause for the episode, e.g. malignancy.

d. Any 2 from: 2 marks
- Perforation.
- Peritonitis.
- Fistula.
- Abscess.
- Bowel obstruction.

e. Any 2 from: 2 marks
- High-fibre diet.
- Weight loss.
- Low-fat diet.
- Increase exercise.

2)

a. An ileus is reduced peristaltic bowel movement which causes features 2 marks
    similar to mechanical obstruction.

b. A plain abdominal X-ray can confirm the diagnosis and will show 2 marks
    dilated small bowel loops.

c. Any 2 from: 2 marks
    ● NG tube insertion.
    ● Nil by mouth.
    ● IV fluids.

d. This patient's ileus should resolve spontaneously over the next few 1 mark
    days. Oral fluids and diet can then be gradually reintroduced.

e. Any 3 from: 3 marks
    ● Adhesions.
    ● Hernia.
    ● Inflammatory bowel disease.
    ● Malignancy.
    ● Volvulus.
    ● Meckel's diverticulum.
    ● Ischaemic colitis.
    ● Intussusception.
    ● Gallstone ileus.

3)

a. Colonoscopy.   1 mark

b. Biopsy during colonoscopy.   2 marks
    CT of the chest, abdomen and pelvis.

c. Epithelium in the colon has a rapid cell turnover. Sporadic genetic 4 marks
    mutations, including activation of oncogenes and inactivation of
    tumour suppressor genes (1 mark), lead to hyperplasia and the
    formation of polyps (adenomas) (1 mark). Further mutation can then
    lead to progression from adenoma to adenocarcinoma (1 mark). If the
    tumour becomes invasive of surrounding tissues, it is an
    adenocarcinoma rather than a benign adenoma (1 mark).

d.   Any 2 from: 2 marks
   ● The screening programme for bowel cancer in the UK is faecal
     occult blood testing for patients aged 60-74 years every 2 years.
   ● Patients send in stool samples which are tested for blood.
     Patients with a positive result are offered a colonoscopy to
     investigate for polyps or malignancy.
   ● Patients under aged 55 years may be offered a one-off bowel
     scope screening test prior to the faecal occult blood testing
     programme.
e.   Left hemicolectomy.   1 mark

4)
a.   Any 2 from: 2 marks
   ● Constipation.
   ● Pregnancy.
   ● Straining.
   ● Ascites.
   ● Chronic cough.
   ● Heavy lifting.
   ● Increased age.
   ● Family history.
b.   Internal haemorrhoids develop above the pectinate line whereas   1 mark
     external haemorrhoids develop below.
c.   Any 2 from: 2 marks
   ● Anal fissure.
   ● Rectal cancer.
   ● Anal cancer.
   ● Rectal polyps.
   ● Diverticular disease.
   ● Inflammatory bowel disease.
   ● Rectal prolapse.
   ● Genital warts.
d.   Any 2 from: 2 marks
   ● High-fibre diet.
   ● Topical corticosteroids.
   ● Analgesia.

e.   Any 3 from: 3 marks
   ● Banding.
   ● Sclerotherapy.
   ● Electrotherapy.
   ● Haemorrhoidal artery ligation.
   ● Haemorrhoidectomy.

5)

a.   Any 2 from: 2 marks
   ● Size of hernia.
   ● Reducibility.
   ● Tenderness.

b.   Incisional hernias occur at a surgical wound site. Separation of the   2 marks
      wound edges allows protrusion of viscus through the abdominal wall
      layers.

c.   Any 3 from: 3 marks
   ● Emergency surgery.
   ● Obesity.
   ● Wound infection.
   ● Poor surgical technique when closing the wound.
   ● Increased intra-abdominal pressure, e.g. chronic cough/ascites,
     etc.
   ● Midline incision.
   ● Older age.
   ● Chemotherapy.
   ● Blood transfusion intra-operatively.

d.   This patient should have a surgical repair — if untreated, the hernia is   1 mark
      likely to enlarge and cause problems.

e.   Any 2 from: 2 marks
   ● Obstruction.
   ● Strangulation.
   ● Ischaemia.
   ● Chronic pain.

6)

a. Any 2 from: 2 marks

- Guarding.
- Rebound tenderness.
- Percussion tenderness.
- Rovsing's sign: pain in the right iliac fossa on palpation of the left iliac fossa.
- Psoas sign: pain on extension of the right hip due to a retrocaecal inflamed appendix coming into contact with the psoas muscle.

b. Appendicitis occurs due to obstruction of the appendiceal lumen, usually due to a faeceolith. This then results in inflammation, which can cause localised peritonitis and may lead to generalised peritonitis if the appendix perforates. 2 marks

c. Emergency appendicectomy. 1 mark

d. Any 2 from: 2 marks

- Malignancy.
- Ulcerative colitis/Crohn's disease.
- Ovarian cyst pathology.
- Pelvic inflammatory disease.
- Renal colic.
- UTI.
- Pyelonephritis.
- Diverticulitis.
- Mesenteric adenitis.
- Inflamed Meckel's diverticulum.
- Testicular torsion.

e. A palpable mass suggests an appendiceal abscess (1 mark). This is treated by an appendicectomy as in uncomplicated appendicitis (1 mark). Antibiotics and a drain are likely to be required to allow for drainage of any intra-abdominal collection (1 mark). 3 marks

7)

a. A pilonidal sinus forms when a hair follicle in the sacrococcygeal region becomes inflamed. The hair grows inwards, forming a 'pit' (1 mark). Debris builds up causing elongation and sinus formation (1 mark). If the sinus becomes infected, an abscess forms (1 mark).   3 marks

b. Antibiotics, e.g. flucloxacillin.   1 mark

c. Incision and drainage.   1 mark

d. Any 3 from: 3 marks
- Male sex.
- Age 15-30 years.
- Obesity.
- Large amounts of hair.
- Caucasian.
- Prolonged sitting.
- Poor hygiene.

e. Any 2 from: 2 marks
- Keeping buttocks clean.
- Losing weight.
- Shaving hair in the affected area.

8)

a. Any 2 from: 2 marks
- Ulcers.
- Pseudopolyps.
- Inflammation of mucosa only.
- Crypt abscesses.
- Reduced goblet cells.
- Continuous inflammation.

b. Any 2 from: 2 marks
- Thumbprinting.
- Mural thickening.
- Mucosal islands.

c.   If the patient does not respond to medical treatment and if any   2 marks
     complications are present.

d.   Any 2 from: 2 marks
     ● Erythema nodosum.
     ● Enteropathic arthritis.
     ● Episcleritis.
     ● Uveitis.
     ● Iritis.
     ● Primary sclerosing cholangitis.

e.   Any 2 from: 2 marks
     ● Toxic megacolon.
     ● Perforation.
     ● Pouchitis.
     ● Dehydration.
     ● Anaemia due to mucosal bleeding.

9)

a.   Any 2 from: 2 marks
     ● Erythema.
     ● Tenderness or warmth surrounding the wound.
     ● Pain.
     ● Wound discharge.
     ● Signs of systemic infection.

b.   Any 2 from: 2 marks
     ● Scrubbing in before surgery.
     ● Use of protective gowns.
     ● Gloves and drapes.
     ● Laminar air flow.
     ● Prophylactic antibiotics.
     ● Skin preparation with antiseptic.
     ● Use of appropriate dressing.

c.   Obesity.   3 marks
     Diabetes.
     Smoking.

d. Any 1 from: 1 mark
    ● Bloods for infection markers.
    ● Blood cultures.
    ● Wound swab.
e. Any 2 from: 2 marks
    ● The patient should be started on appropriate antibiotics.
    ● Staples or sutures should be removed to allow pus drainage.
    ● The wound can be packed if needed.

10)
a. Any 2 from: 2 marks
    ● Site in right iliac fossa.
    ● Spouted to stop damage to the skin from contents.
    ● Contents of bag mainly liquid.
b. Any 2 from: 2 marks
    ● Jejunostomy.
    ● Urostomy.
    ● Colostomy.
c. Any 2 from: 2 marks
    ● IV fluids.
    ● Replace electrolytes.
    ● Antimotility medication.
d. Any 2 from: 2 marks
    ● Prolapse.
    ● Stenosis.
    ● Parastomal hernia.
    ● Mucocutaneous separation.
    ● Trauma.
    ● Necrosis.
    ● Retraction.
e. Any 2 from: 2 marks
    ● Pale colour (anaemia).
    ● Dusky colour (ischaemia).

- Ribbon-like stools (stenosis).
- Abnormal appearance of surrounding skin, e.g. erythema/rash.
- Separation of the mucocutaneous junction.

11)

a. Any 2 from: 2 marks
- Generalised tenderness.
- Guarding.
- Peritonism.
- Abdominal distention.
- Features of shock.

b. Any 3 from: 3 marks
- Peptic ulcer.
- Malignancy.
- inflammatory bowel disease.
- Ischaemic colitis.
- Infection.
- Surgery/endoscopy.
- Trauma.
- Vomiting (Boerhaave syndrome).

c. Erect chest X-ray (shows air under the diaphragm confirming a 1 mark pneumoperitoneum).

d. This patient needs IV antibiotics (1 mark) and to be taken to theatre 2 marks for washout and repair or resection of the affected part of the bowel (1 mark). Patients with localised perforations may be managed conservatively but this patient has systemic features of sepsis.

e. Any 2 from: 2 marks
- The junction between the pharynx and oesophagus.
- The oesophagus at the level of the aortic arch.
- Lower oesophageal sphincter.
- Pylorus of the stomach.
- Curvature of the duodenum.
- Ileocaecal valve.

- Hepatic flexure.
- Splenic flexure.

12)

a. Any 4 from: 4 marks
- Previous thrombus.
- Previous emboli.
- Arrhythmias.
- Shock.
- Trauma.
- Strangulated hernia.
- Strangulated volvulus.
- Recent surgery.
- Vasculitic disease.
- Sickle cell disease.
- Coagulopathic disease.
- Digitalis.
- Oestrogens.
- Antihypertensives.
- Cocaine.
- Vasopressin.
- Phenylephrine.
- Immunosuppressants.
- Psychotropic agents.

b. Watershed areas where there are anastomoses between different 1 mark arterial supplies (1 mark), such as the distal third of the transverse colon.

c. From the second part of the duodenum up to and including the 2 marks proximal two thirds of the transverse colon.

d. Any 2 from: 2 marks
- Fluid resuscitation.
- Antibiotics.
- Nil by mouth.
- NG tube

e.   Resection of the affected bowel and stoma formation if necessary.   1 mark

13)

a.   Volvulus is the twisting of a section of bowel on its mesentery, leading   1 mark
to obstruction and potentially ischaemia.

b.   Sigmoid colon. On X-ray this gives a 'coffee bean sign' — a dilated loop   2 marks
of bowel arising in the left iliac fossa.

c.   Any 2 from: 2 marks
- Neuropsychiatric disorders.
- Male sex.
- Diabetes.
- Chronic constipation.
- Increased age.
- Nursing home resident.
- History of abdominal surgery.

d.   Insertion of a flatus tube via a sigmoidoscope.   3 marks
Any 2 from:
- Surgical management is required if multiple attempts at a flatus
  tube fail.
- Perforation.
- Peritonitis.
- Necrosis.

e.   Any 2 from: 2 marks
- Gangrenous bowel.
- Ischaemia.
- Perforation.
- Recurrence.

Chapter 12

Vascular surgery
ANSWERS

Single best answers

1) c.
2) b.
3) b.
4) c.
5) a.
6) a.
7) d.
8) d.
9) c.
10) a.
11) c.
12) b.
13) c.
14) a.
15) a.
16) a.
17) c.
18) c.
19) b.
20) a.

21) d.
22) d.
23) c.

Extended matching question answers

1) c

An ABPI of less than 0.4 is seen in critical limb ischaemia and is defined as rest pain which is present for over 2 weeks with or without ulceration or gangrene. A value of less than 0.3 implies impending gangrene.

2) g

An ABPI of greater than 1.3 is strongly suggestive of incompressible and calcified arterial walls which occurs in renal failure or diabetes mellitus.

3) f

A normal range for the ABPI is between 0.9 and 1.1; values less than this indicate arterial disease.

4) e

An ABPI value of between 0.7 and 0.9 indicates mild arterial disease which can present as mild claudication.

5) d

An ABPI value of between 0.4 and 0.7 indicates moderate arterial disease which can present as severe claudication.

6) c

Leriche syndrome is a triad of claudication of the buttock/thighs, absent femoral pulses and erectile dysfunction. It is caused by blockage of the abdominal aorta as it becomes the common iliac arteries. It is also known as aortoiliac occlusive disease.

7) e

Lipodermatosclerosis is characterised by eczema, itching fat necrosis and pigmentation. It is associated with chronic venous insufficiency. The brown pigment is haemosiderin deposition from red blood cells.

8) f

This patient is presenting with the classical signs of DVT. She would score 4 on the Wells score. Virchow's triad highlights the predisposing factors for thrombus formation which are venous stasis, endothelial damage and a hypercoagulable state.

9) b

Critical limb ischaemia is defined as rest pain which is present for over 2 weeks with or without ulceration or gangrene.

10) d

A patient with known AF presenting with signs of an acutely ischaemic limb should prompt the clinician to rule out an embolic cause of the symptoms. Acute limb ischaemia is a surgical emergency and requires treatment within 6 hours of symptoms occurring.

11) a

The patient is describing the classical symptoms of Raynaud's syndrome. In this case, it is caused by a cervical rib which is an additional rib arising from the seventh cervical vertebrae above the first rib. This additional structure causes compression on the vasculature and nervous structures that traverse the surface of the first rib leading to symptoms.

12) d

ACE inhibitors are contraindicated in renal artery stenosis. In this condition, renal perfusion is reduced resulting in hypertension. The afferent pressure is reduced by the stenosed vessel so the process of autoregulation is dependent on the efferent limb. If ACE inhibitors are used, the renin-angiotensin system is disrupted resulting in impaired autoregulation leading to a fall in GFR and renal ischaemia causing renal failure.

13) g

This patient has a Stanford Type A dissection that requires surgical intervention. A Stanford Type A dissection involves the ascending aorta or aortic arch whilst a Type B dissection involves the descending aorta distal to the left subclavian artery, which can be treated with medical therapy through control of hypertension.

14) c

Subclavian steal syndrome is due to proximal subclavian artery stenosis or occlusion which leads to retrograde vertebral artery flow in order to preserve the affected limb blood supply which results in cerebral ischaemia and the neurological symptoms experienced by the patient.

15) e

The most common cause of secondary lymphoedema is filariasis which is caused by *Wuchereria bancrofti*. It is transmitted by mosquitos resulting in lymphadenopathy, fever, inguinal pain and limb swelling.

16) g

Duplex ultrasound is the preferred imaging method for patients with varicose veins following a DVT. It helps to map the source and course of the varicosities and ensure that the deep venous system is intact.

17) d

Any elderly patient who has vague abdominal pain who has a history of vascular disease should be screened for an abdominal aortic aneurysm as the cause of their pain.

18) e

The patient has a previous history of DVT and coupled with the shortness of breath and sinus tachycardia would raise the suspicion of a pulmonary embolism which can be assessed using CTPA.

19) c

The patient has an arterial ulcer and the ABPI will be reduced in this patient reflecting arterial disease.

20) g

Colour duplex ultrasound is the gold standard for evaluating carotid artery stenosis as a cause for a patient's TIA symptoms.

21) b

A reperfusion injury can occur if the limb has been ischaemic for a long period of time with areas of significant muscle damage. Restoring the blood supply to this area releases a wave of toxins into the systemic circulation including potassium and myoglobin which can cause cardiovascular collapse, renal failure and acute respiratory distress syndrome.

22) f

An endoleak is a consequence of an endovascular repair procedure in which the graft fails to completely seal the aneurysm allowing blood to leak back into the aneurysm sac.

23) g

Compartment syndrome is a life- and limb-threatening emergency that requires prompt treatment. It develops due to an increased pressure in a closed tissue space such as a muscle compartment. This increased pressure compromises blood flow. A high index of suspicion is needed and any patient who has pain that does not fit with the clinical picture should be assessed for compartment syndrome.

24) c

The patient has experienced spinal cord ischaemia which has led to paralysis. It is a complication of aortic aneurysm surgery and it is thought to be due to the loss of the artery of Adamkiewicz which is responsible for supplying the distal two thirds of the spinal cord. The artery of Adamkiewicz is a branch of the thoracic aorta and supplies the spinal cord by the anterior spinal artery.

25) h

Graft infection can present many years after the initial procedure and requires a combination of antibiotic therapy and removal of the graft.

26) e

This patient scores for having major surgery in the past 4 weeks (1), calf swelling >3cm compared with the other leg (1), the entire leg is swollen (1), and pitting oedema is confirmed in the symptomatic leg (1).

27) d

This patient scores for the presence of collateral (non-varicose) superficial veins (1), the entire leg is swollen (1) and he has a previously documented DVT (1).

28) a

This patient scores for swelling of the entire leg (1); however, as a diagnosis of cellulitis is more likely in this case, she loses 2 points for an alternative diagnosis being more likely than DVT (-2).

29) f

This patient scores for active cancer treatment (1), calf swelling >3cm compared with the other side (1), the entire leg is swollen (1), localised tenderness along the deep venous system (1) and pitting oedema is confirmed in the symptomatic leg (1).

30) c

This patient scores for calf swelling >3cm compared with the other side (1) and recent plaster immobilisation of the lower extremity (1).

31) a

This patient has a non-viable limb and therefore it must be removed. If the limb was reperfused, there is a high risk of a reperfusion injury.

32) e

This patient has acute limb ischaemia secondary to an embolism due to his AF. Embolectomy aims to remove the emboli that is blocking the circulation and restoring blood flow to the area.

33) b

This patient has intermittent claudication. The first-line management is to encourage a healthy diet, weight loss and control of comorbidities and risk factors such as hypertension, diabetes, cholesterol and smoking. If the patient's symptoms continued to deteriorate and he developed critical limb ischaemia, surgery could be considered.

34) g

A femoral-popliteal bypass can be used to bypass stenosis in the superficial femoral artery. Bypass surgery is best used in multilevel disease or long occlusions.

35) d

The patient has a compartment syndrome and the pressure must be reduced by an urgent fasciotomy.

36) b

A venous ulcer is commonly located on the gaiter region above the medial malleolus and is shallow, irregular and has a base of granulation tissue. The skin around the site may demonstrate venous changes and distal pulses will be present. The ABPI is usually normal.

37) c

A neuropathic ulcer is located at points of high pressure including the dorsum of the toes and plantar aspects of the metatarsal heads or heel. It is usually a deep ulceration with well-defined edges. The cuff of callous indicates an area of repeated trauma. The foot is usually warm and the ABPI is normal unless there is other peripheral arterial disease.

38) a

An arterial ulcer is usually located on the dorsum on the foot but it can occur anywhere. The lesions are small with a well-circumscribed border and appear punched out. They have a poorly healing base with a delayed capillary refill time. Distal pulses are absent and the ABPI is less than 0.5.

39) g

A Marjolin ulcer is the development of a squamous cell carcinoma in the site of a scar or ulcer. They behave aggressively and can metastasise to lymph nodes.

40) f

A Curling's ulcer or stress ulcer is due to acute gastric erosion resulting from complication of severe burns where the reduced plasma volume results in ischaemia and necrosis of gastric mucosa leading to ulceration.

41) a

AAAs that are between 4cm and 5.5cm and are asymptomatic should be rescanned every 6 months.

42) f

This patient has a ruptured AAA that requires immediate repair. The patient should be taken to the operating theatre following stabilisation. If the patient was not stable or the diagnosis was not in doubt, then a CT should not be performed and they should be taken straight to theatre.

43) e

An increase of >1cm per year is an indication for an urgent elective repair.

44) h

Endovascular repair is suitable for AAAs that begin 3cm below the renal arteries. A graft is passed into the femoral artery and passed into the aorta where it is deployed to seal the aneurysm sac and reduce the pressure burden on the diseased section of aortic wall.

45) b

If an AAA is less than 4cm and the patient is asymptomatic, then the patient can be screened annually for changes in size. Treatment options and follow-up can be arranged accordingly.

Short answer question answers

a. Critical limb ischaemia. 1 mark

b. Any 2 from: 2 marks

- Critical limb ischaemia is defined as rest pain which is present for over 2 weeks with or without ulceration or gangrene.
- It is often worst at night.
- It can be improved by hanging the leg out of bed.

c. Any 4 from: 2 marks

- Smoking.
- Diabetes.
- Hypercholesterolaemia.
- Hypertension.
- Cardiovascular disease.
- Family history of hyperhomocysteinaemia.

d. Any 2 from: 2 marks

- ECG.
- ABPI.
- Duplex Doppler.
- Arteriography.
- Magnetic resonance angiogram.

e. Any 3 from: 3 marks

- Angioplasty.
- Stenting.
- Bypass grafting.
- Amputation.

2)

a. Any 4 from: 2 marks
- Atherosclerosis.
- Marfan syndrome.
- Ehlers-Danlos syndrome.
- Abdominal trauma.
- Tertiary syphilis.
- *Salmonella typhi.*
- *Escherichia coli.*
- Inflammation.
- Post-stenosis.

b. Any 2 from: 2 marks
- True aneurysm.
- False aneurysm.
- Fusiform aneurysm.
- Saccular aneurysm.

c. Any 4 from: 2 marks
- Aneurysm diameter ≥5.5cm.
- Aneurysm increasing by ≥1cm per year.
- Symptomatic aneurysm.
- Thromboembolic event due to aneurysm.
- Rupture.

d. All males over 65 years (1 mark) are offered an ultrasound and if 2 marks normal require no further imaging. Aneurysms between 3-4.4cm receive yearly screening whilst aneurysms between 4.4-5.4cm receive 3-monthly screening. Aneurysms greater than 5.5cm are referred for elective repair consideration (1 mark).

e. Any 2 from: 2 marks
- Intracranial (Berry aneurysm).
- Popliteal artery.
- Femoral artery.
- Iliac artery.

3)

a. Any 2 symptoms from: 2 marks
- Calf pain.
- Stiffness.
- Fever.

Any 2 signs from:
- Unilateral leg swelling.
- Calf tenderness.
- Warm skin.
- Dilated superficial veins.

b. Endothelial injury: trauma, surgery, atherosclerosis, venepuncture, 3 marks cardiac valve disease.

Stasis of blood flow: AF, left ventricular dysfunction, immobility, varicose veins.

Hypercoagulability: malignancy, pregnancy, oestrogen therapy, sepsis, thrombophilia.

c. Wells score of 5. This patient scores for active cancer treatment (1), 1 mark calf swelling >3cm compared with the other side (1), the entire leg is swollen (1), localised tenderness along the deep venous system (1) and pitting oedema is confirmed in the symptomatic leg (1).

d. Any 1 from: 1 mark
- Low-molecular-weight heparin.
- Warfarin.
- Direct oral anticoagulants, e.g. rivaroxaban, apixaban, dabigatran.

e. Any 3 from: 3 marks
- Pulmonary embolism.
- Leg pain.
- Leg swelling.
- Itching.
- Skin discolouration.
- Leg ulcers.
- Post-thrombotic syndrome.

4)

a. Any 3 from: 3 marks
   - Arterial.
   - Venous.
   - Neuropathic.
   - Pressure.

b. Any 2 from: 2 marks
   - Duplex Doppler ultrasound.
   - Wound swab.
   - Bloods including FBC and U&Es.

c. Any 3 from: 3 marks
   - Varicose veins.
   - Lipodermatosclerosis.
   - Haemosiderin deposition.
   - Varicose eczema.
   - Lymphoedema.
   - Thickened skin.
   - Papillomatosis.
   - Fissuring.
   - Hyperkeratosis.

d. Compression bandaging.   1 mark

e. Marjolin ulcer.   1 mark

5)

a. Any 4 from: 2 marks
   - Thrombosis: atherosclerosis, popliteal aneurysm, bypass-graft occlusion, thrombotic conditions.
   - Embolism: AF, mural thrombosis, vegetation, proximal aneurysm, atherosclerotic plaque rupture.
   - Other: dissection, trauma, external compression, compartment syndrome.

b. Pain.   3 marks
   Pallor.

Perishing cold.

Paraesthesia.

Paralysis.

Pulselessness.

c. Any 2 from: 1 mark

- ECG.
- Duplex Doppler.
- Arteriography.
- ABG.

d. Any 1 from: 1 mark

- Thrombolysis.
- Embolectomy.
- Angioplasty.
- Arterial bypass grafting.

e. Viable: Doppler pulses present, limb not immediately threatened,   3 marks
sensation intact.

Threatened: loss of sensory and motor function, urgent treatment
required.

Irreversible: fixed mottling with muscle paralysis, requires
amputation.

6)

a. Any 2 symptoms from: 4 marks

- Severe sudden-onset retrosternal chest pain.
- Tearing pain.
- Pain radiating to the back and arms.
- Shortness of breath.
- Nausea.
- Vomiting.
- Syncope.
- Abdominal pain.
- Paralysis.

Any 2 signs from:

- Shock.
- Oliguria.
- Hypertension.
- Fever.
- Absence of peripheral pulses.
- Asymmetrical peripheral pulses.
- Diastolic murmur in keeping with aortic regurgitation.

b. Any 2 from: 1 mark
- Hypertension.
- Trauma.
- Marfan syndrome.
- Ehlers-Danlos syndrome.
- Syphilis.
- Vasculitis.
- Medial degeneration.

c. Stanford Classification: Type I is an intimal tear in the ascending aorta   2 marks
and descending aorta. Type II is confined to the ascending aorta. Type
III is confined to the descending aorta only.
De Bakey Classification: Type A dissection affects the ascending aorta.
Type B dissection affects the descending aorta.

d. Any 2 from: 2 marks
- ECG.
- Chest X-ray.
- CT scan.
- Angiography.
- Aortography.
- Transoesophageal echo.

e. Aggressive medical management of blood pressure is indicated for a   1 mark
Stanford Type B dissection unless there is a rupture or lower limb
ischaemia.

7)

a. Any 2 from: 2 marks

- Direct pressure on the wound.
- Elevate limb.
- Urgent vascular review.
- Tourniquet.

b. Any 3 from: 3 marks

- Femoral artery.
- Femoral vein.
- Femoral nerve.
- Lymphatic system.

c. Any 2 from: 2 marks

- Bruit.
- Active haemorrhage.
- Pulsatile haemorrhage.
- Haematoma formation.
- Pain.
- Paralysis.
- Paraesthesia.
- Pallor.
- Perishing cold.
- Pulselessness.
- Hypotension.
- Proximity of injury to vascular structures.

d. Any 1 from: 1 mark

- Vein patch in a longitudinal arteriotomy.
- Primary closure in a transverse arteriotomy.

e. Any 2 from: 2 marks

- Ischaemia.
- Necrosis.
- Gangrene.
- Ischaemic contracture.
- Pseudoaneurysm.
- Amputation.

8)

a.   AAA rupture.   1 mark

b.   Any 6 from: 3 marks
   ● Administer high-flow oxygen.
   ● Vascular access.
   ● ABG.
   ● Bloods including FBC, U&Es, clotting, group and save.
   ● Fluid resuscitation using crystalloids or blood products.
   ● Analgesia.
   ● Catheterisation.
   ● Urgent vascular review and anaesthetic review.
   ● CT of the thorax/abdomen if the patient is stable.
   ● ECG.

c.   Permissive hypotension is a strategy used in the resuscitation of   2 marks
      bleeding trauma patients. This advocates the cautious use of fluid to
      maintain a blood pressure lower than normal but that can sustain
      sufficient organ perfusion. It is believed to prevent a large increase in
      blood pressure to disrupt clot formation, avoid further tearing to the
      aorta and limit blood loss.

d.   The most common procedure is an urgent open repair using an in-lay   2 marks
      graft such as a Dacron® graft or some centres are now trialling
      endovascular repair.

e.   Any 2 from: 2 marks
   ● Haemorrhage.
   ● Ischaemic leg.
   ● Trash foot.
   ● Myocardial infarction.
   ● Renal failure.
   ● DIC.
   ● ARDS.
   ● Colonic ischaemia.
   ● Pneumonia.
   ● Stroke.

- DVT.
- PE.
- Spinal ischaemia leading to paraparesis.
- Graft infection.
- Aorto-enteric fistula.

9)

a. Classified as primary which is the degeneration of the valve annulus 2 marks
and leaflets; and secondary which is due to valve destruction or
venous outflow destruction.

b. Any 2 from: 2 marks
- Female.
- Pregnancy.
- Pelvic mass.
- Abdominal mass.
- Previous DVT.
- Family history.
- Obesity.
- Occupations involving long periods of standing.

c. Any 2 from: 2 marks
- Long saphenous-femoral vein junction.
- Short saphenous-popliteal vein junction.
- Perforating veins.

d. Any 3 from: 3 marks
- No treatment.
- Watchful waiting.
- Leg elevation.
- Graduation compression stockings.
- Sclerotherapy.
- Ligation and stripping.
- Endovenous laser ablation.
- Endoluminal radiofrequency ablation.
- Foam injection.

e. Delay surgery until after completed family, as pregnancy is a risk   1 mark
    factor for reoccurrence.

10)

a. Any 4 from: 4 marks
    - Asymptomatic.
    - Stroke.
    - TIA.
    - Amaurosis fugax.

b. Any 2 from: 2 marks
    - Atherosclerosis of the internal carotid origin (1 mark) leading to
      stenosis (1 mark).
    - Unstable plaques may form (1 mark), which are a source of
      cerebral circulation emboli (1 mark).

c. Any 1 from: 1 mark
    - Duplex ultrasound.
    - Magnetic resonance angiography.
    - CT scan.
    - Angiography.

d. Carotid endarterectomy. Angioplasty or stenting are not acceptable   1 mark
    as these are reserved for previous surgery or radiotherapy.

e. Any 4 from: 2 marks
    - Smoking cessation.
    - Regular physical activity.
    - Dietary changes.
    - Control hypertension.
    - Good glycaemic control.
    - Statin therapy.
    - Antiplatelet therapy.

11)

a. Atherosclerosis.   4 marks
    Infection.

Impaired tissue metabolism.

Peripheral neuropathy.

b. Any 4 from: 2 marks
- Sensory neuropathy.
- Altered foot shape.
- Ill-fitting shoes.
- Previous ulceration.
- Increasing age.
- Peripheral vascular disease.
- Visual impairment.
- Living alone.

c. Any 4 from: 2 marks
- Regular self-examination.
- Regular medical review.
- Pressure relief.
- Chiropody.
- Wearing appropriate shoes.
- Avoiding potential damage.
- Avoiding heat sources.

d. Any 2 from: 1 mark
- Good glycaemic control.
- Control of cholesterol.
- Antiplatelet agents.
- Control of hypertension.

e. Arteries may be highly calcified which leads to reduced elasticity 1 mark
resulting in stiff arteries and falsely elevated ankle pressures.

12)
a. Compartment syndrome.   1 mark
b. Any 4 from: 2 marks
- Fractures.
- Crush injury.
- Revascularisation.

- Bleeding.
- Burns.
- Severe shock.
- Overly tight bandaging or plaster.
- Prolonged compression.
- Surgery to blood vessels in arms or legs.
- Blood clots.
- Extremely vigorous exercise.

c. Any 3 early signs from: 3 marks
- Pain out of proportion to injury.
- Pain on stretching of affected muscle groups.
- Absent distal pulse.
- Markedly swollen area.

Any 3 late signs from:
- Paralysis.
- Weakness.
- Pale limb.
- Cold limb.
- Sensory loss.

d. Any 2 from: 2 marks
- Split plaster/bandages.
- Compartment pressures if diagnosis in doubt.
- Urgent fasciotomy.

e. Any 2 from: 2 marks
- Muscle wasting.
- Nerve injury.
- Foot drop.
- Muscle fibrosis.
- Claw toes.
- Joint dislocation.
- Cavus deformity.
- Sensory neuropathy.

13)

a. Primary lymphoedema occurs due to a developmental abnormality of   2 marks
    the lymphatic system. Secondary lymphoedema is a result of
    obstruction or damage to the lymphatic system.

b. Any 2 primary causes: 2 marks
    - Congenital.
    - Idiopathic.
    - Milroy's disease.
    - Lymphoedema praecox.
    - Lymphoedema tarda.

    Any 2 secondary causes:
    - Groin surgery.
    - Axillary surgery.
    - Post-radiotherapy.
    - Malignancy.
    - Filariasis.
    - Lymphadenectomy.
    - Chronic inflammation.

c. Any 2 from: 2 marks
    - Venous oedema.
    - Cardiac failure.
    - Hepatic insufficiency.
    - Hypoproteinaemia.
    - Renal failure.
    - Gravitational oedema.
    - Stasis.
    - Post-phlebitic oedema.

d. Lymphoscintigraphy: a delayed transit of injected dye into   2 marks
    subcutaneous tissue confirms the diagnosis of lymphoedema.
    Lymphangiography: delineates anatomy prior to surgery.

e. Any 2 from: 2 marks
    - Limb elevation.
    - Compression bandaging.

- Stocking.
- Pneumatic compression.
- Antibiotics to treat infections.
- Exclude other treatable causes of oedema.
- Surgery.

(Note: diuretics do not reduce lymphoedema!)

Chapter 13

Breast surgery
ANSWERS

Single best answers

1) d.
2) c.
3) b.
4) b.
5) a.
6) d.
7) d.
8) a.
9) c.
10) c.
11) b.
12) d.
13) b.
14) a.
15) a.
16) a.
17) d.
18) c.
19) d.
20) a.

21) c.
22) b.
23) b.

Extended matching question answers

1) c

 This is a classic presentation of lactational mastitis and sepsis should be considered.

2) e

 Lipomas are common and can occur anywhere on the body. This patient is young and the lump is described as superficial. There are no worrying features in the history. If there were any concerns, a referral to dermatology/breast services would be appropriate.

3) f

 In breast abscesses there is usually a recent history of mastitis. The abscess can cause pain, swelling and skin changes.

4) h

 Breast cysts often develop over the age of 35 and around the time of menopause. They can be multiple and of any size. They are more often incidental findings during breast screening and depending on their position they can be aspirated.

5) b

 Breast cancer. This is a description of "Paget's disease of the nipple". It can be a sign of underlying breast cancer and should be investigated via a 2-week wait/urgent referral. Investigations usually involve a mammogram/USS and punch biopsy.

6)   a

Lobular breast cancer cannot always be seen on a mammogram and often does not present with a lump. In such cases, the cancer can be invasive by the time it is diagnosed.

7)   c

The UK screening program consists of mammogram imaging.

8)   f

Most women under 40 will undergo an ultrasound scan as the imaging modality of choice. This is due to increased breast density.

9)   b

This patient may have a breast cancer that has metastasised to her brain. Confused elderly patients can be difficult to assess. In this case, a CT of the head should be carried out to look for intracranial pathology and if lesions are seen then investigations for the primary cancer must be carried out.

10)   b

This patient is likely to have a PE. She would score over 4 points on Wells' PE scoring system as she has no signs/symptoms to suggest another cause.

11)   h

The intercostobrachial nerve supplies sensation to the axilla. It is often sacrificed during breast surgery.

12)   e

The thoracodorsal nerve is usually located and protected during breast surgery. It supplies the latissimus dorsi muscle which is responsible for the above movements.

13) a

The axillary nerve can be stretched after anterior dislocation of the shoulder joint. It is important to document axillary nerve function both before and after relocation.

14) g

The radial nerve travels in the radial groove of the humerus. It is at this point that it is vulnerable to damage during mid-shaft fractures.

15) b

This patient has likely had an axillary node clearance with long thoracic nerve damage. The nerve supplies serratus anterior which stabilises the scapula. Damage to this nerve results in 'winging'.

16) d

Tamoxifen is given to premenopausal women with oestrogen-positive disease. It acts as an antagonist in breast tissue but an agonist in the endometrium so any symptoms of abnormal vaginal bleeding must be fully investigated.

17) e

These agents are suitable for postmenopausal women as they only affect oestrogen made in the peripheries (not ovaries) so this would not be recommended for premenopausal women.

18) c

Herceptin® (trastuzumab) is a treatment that can be used for HER 2-positive breast cancers.

19) b

Triple-negative disease will not respond to the respective therapies and is therefore more difficult to treat and can be more aggressive.

20) c

Herceptin® (trastuzumab) is a treatment that can be used for HER 2-positive breast cancers.

21) b

Anyone aged 50 or over with unilateral nipple symptoms should be referred urgently as it may be a sign of underlying breast cancer.

22) a

A thorough family history must be taken. This patient has one first and one second-degree relative with breast cancer warranting routine referral.

23) f

This patient likely has cyclical breast pain. In order to assess this, patients are asked to keep a diary of their menstrual cycle and their pain for 2 months. They should then be seen again by their primary care doctor to confirm the cause and offer appropriate advice.

24) g

This patient has sepsis secondary to mastitis. Although she will need to be seen by the breast team at some point, the most appropriate first step is to send her to the emergency department. She is haemodynamically unstable (low BP) and needs immediate management.

25) b

Anyone over the age of 30 with an unexplained breast lump should be referred for urgent assessment.

26) b

This is suspicious of lymphadenopathy. Anyone over 30 years of age with an axillary lump should be referred urgently. These nodes could be reactive or cancer-related. This includes breast and other cancers, e.g. melanoma. They need further assessment to establish the cause.

27) a

Patients under the age of 30 with breast lumps can be reviewed by the breast team in a routine manner as these are much more likely to be benign in origin.

28) a

Anyone with a first-degree male relative diagnosed with breast cancer (at any age) can be referred to secondary care.

29) d

Under current guidance there is no indication for secondary care involvement as this patient's mother is over the age of 40 and does not carry any increased risk factors, e.g. ovarian cancer. She can be reassured that there is currently no need for concern; however, she should be advised to return if she notices any breast changes, or if the family history changes.

30) a

If patients are not reassured by primary care and still have concerns, they can be referred to a breast clinic to discuss this.

31) g

These usually present over the age of 40 once the breast starts to age. They can produce blood-stained or clear discharge and can also be painless. They still require triple assessment as in rare cases they can contain atypical cells.

32) b

This patient most likely has an area of fat necrosis due to trauma from her seatbelt. She would still need to be assessed in the breast clinic to rule out other pathology.

33) c

The patient most likely has duct ectasia. She is close to the age of menopause when ducts shorten and widen.

34) d

This patient most likely has intertrigo from chafing. It can present anywhere where skin rubs onto skin, which becomes difficult to keep dry.

35) a

This patient has thrombophlebitis following biopsy. This can cause pain and redness and with time the cord-like structure becomes firm and can pucker the skin.

36) c

The most likely problem is a haematoma from a bleeding vessel. The swelling can be extensive and painful. The mild tachycardia is secondary to the acute bleeding. Haematomas usually need to be drained if large to stop bleeding and protect skin integrity.

37) b

Allergic reactions can present with classical symptoms of wheeze, rash and fainting but can also present with diarrhoea, vomiting and abdominal pain. It is likely she has been prescribed a painkiller, given her history of asthma; this could be NSAID-related.

38) g

This patient has a seroma. These do not tend to collect immediately after surgery so people notice them over the coming weeks. This mastectomy with axillary node clearance provides a potential space for fluid to accumulate. Unlike an abscess/cellulitis, patients are usually well, and symptoms relate to size and pressure on surrounding structures.

39) e

This patient has cellulitis secondary to the skin break caused by the biopsy. She needs oral antibiotics and follow-up to ensure this improves and does not develop into an abscess. Eczema tends to be drier, and abscesses take longer to collect.

40) b

This patient has suffered anaphylaxis to her chemotherapy agent. The quick succession of events points to this. She will need immediate management by the cardiac arrest team.

41) d

This patient's symptoms are consistent with high levels of prolactin. Other symptoms include deranged periods and infertility.

42) e

This patient is in the correct age range for duct ectasia. As women age, the breast secretions build up as ducts shorten and widen.

43) b

These tumours are rare but can present very rapidly and can be very large. They can be benign or malignant and are very aggressive. These patients require regular follow-up as they can regrow after removal.

44) g

Breast screening can detect tumours before they become invasive and are therefore more likely to be curable; they also require less extensive surgery.

45) h

This patient most likely has skin metastasis from recurrent breast cancer. She will need full assessment of the extent of the disease to guide future management.

Short answer question answers

1)

a. Any 2 from: 2 marks
- Lung.
- Prostate.
- GI tract.

b. Any 5 from: 4 marks
- Weakness.
- Brisk reflexes.
- Increased tone.
- Spasticity.
- Clonus.
- Positive Babinski reflex.

c. Steroids, e.g. dexamethasone.   1 mark

d. MRI spine.   1 mark

e. Radiotherapy.   2 marks
Surgery.

2)

a. X-ray.   1 mark

b. Any 6 from: 3 marks
- Fatigue.
- Skin changes.
- Hair loss.
- Gastrointestinal symptoms.
- Low blood counts.
- Pneumonitis.
- Fatigue.
- Sore throat.
- Pain at site of radiotherapy.

c.   Any 6 from: 3 marks
  - Lymphoedema.
  - Delayed healing.
  - Chronic skin changes.
  - Cardiovascular events.
  - A second cancer.
  - Lymphoedema.
  - Osteoporosis.
  - Neurological signs.

d.   Lymphoedema.   1 mark

e.   Ultrasound scan to rule out upper limb DVT.   2 marks

3)

a.   Hypercalcaemia.   1 mark

b.   Hyponatraemia.   4 marks
      Hypokalaemia.
      Metabolic alkalosis from loss of bicarbonate.
      Hypochloraemia.

c.   IV fluids.   1 mark

d.   Catheter insertion to monitor urine output.   2 marks

e.   Bisphosphonates. They work by inhibiting osteoclast activity. 2 marks

4)

a.   Any 6 from: 3 marks
  - Routine bloods.
  - Blood cultures.
  - ECG.
  - Chest X-ray.
  - Urinalysis.
  - Blood gas.
  - Lactate.

b.   Fluids.   3 marks

      Antibiotics.

      Blood cultures.

      Catheter.

      Lactate.

      Oxygen.

c.   Neutropenia.   1 mark

d.   Haematology.   1 mark

e.   Yes. Although it is preferable for patients and their families to be   2 marks
informed about this, it is not a legal requirement.

5)

a.   Pleural effusion.   2 marks

b.   Chest X-ray.   2 marks

c.   A meniscus obscuring the costophrenic angle.   2 marks

d.   Pleural aspiration.   2 marks

e.   Any 2 from: 2 marks

- Exudate.
- Low glucose.
- High protein.
- pH <7.2.
- Raised LDH.
- Normal Gram staining.

6)

a.   Deep vein thrombosis.   1 mark

b.   Any 5 from: 5 marks

- Cellulitis.
- Superficial thrombophlebitis.
- Achilles tendonitis.
- Muscle strain.
- Soft tissue injury.
- Stress fracture.

- Arterial insufficiency.
- Varicose veins.
- Dependent oedema.
- Lymphoedema.

c. Wells score for DVT.   1 mark
d. Ultrasound Doppler.   1 mark
e. Treatment dose of low-molecular-weight heparin.   2 marks
    Analgesia.

7)

a. Proximal fracture of the femur.   1 mark
b. Shortened and externally rotated leg.   3 marks
    Minimal movement of limb.
c. Bony metastasis causing a pathological fracture.   2 marks
d. Orthopaedics; patients with advanced cancer should still be   1 mark
    considered for surgical intervention to help improve pain and quality
    of life.
e. Bisphosphonates.   3 marks
    Denosumab.
    Radiotherapy.

8)

a. Superior vena cava obstruction.   1 mark
b. Any 4 from: 4 marks
    - Stridor.
    - Prominent veins on the chest wall.
    - Oedema in the neck and arms.
    - Engorged face.
    - Difficulty breathing.
    - Dyspnoea.
    - Swollen face.
    - Swollen arms.

c. Lift arms above their head.   1 mark

d. Airway, breathing, circulation, disability, exposure.   1 mark

e. Radiotherapy.   3 marks
    Chemotherapy.
    Stenting.

9)

a. Low-molecular-weight heparin.   1 mark

b. Before, as this is the most likely cause of her symptoms and is   2 marks
    potentially life-threatening. Imaging can take time to organise so
    would delay treatment.

c. By binding to antithrombin inhibiting factor X, therefore disrupting   3 marks
    the clotting cascade.

d. No; however, patients should be monitored for heparin-induced   2 marks
    thrombocytopaenia.

e. Weight.   2 marks
    VTE risk assessment.

10)

a. Any 6 from: 3 marks
    - FBC.
    - B_{12}.
    - Folate.
    - Vitamin D.
    - Calcium.
    - Thyroid-stimulating hormone.
    - Glucose.

b. Depression.   1 mark

c. Any 2 from: 2 marks
    - Patient Health Questionnaire (PHQ-9).
    - Hospital Anxiety and Depression Scale (HADS).
    - Beck Depression Inventory (BDI).

d.   SSRI.   2 marks

   Any 1 from:
   - Citalopram.
   - Escitalopram.
   - Fluoxetine.
   - Fluvoxamine.
   - Paroxetine.
   - Sertraline.

e.   Any suicidal thoughts or suicide plans.   2 marks

11)

a.   *Staphylococcus aureus.*   2 marks

b.   Flucloxacillin.   2 marks

c.   No. You are unsure of the reaction and there are alternatives to 2 marks
   penicillins that can be used safely.

d.   Macrolides.   2 marks

e.   Blood cultures.   2 marks
   Wound swab.

12)

a.   Any 6 from: 3 marks
   - Female.
   - Increasing age.
   - Genetic mutation.
   - Nulliparous.
   - Early menarche.
   - Late menopause.
   - HRT.
   - Chest irradiation (e.g. CT scans).
   - Family history.
   - Previous breast cancer.

b.   Any 4 from: 2 marks
- Firm mass.
- Painless.
- Fixed.
- Nipple inversion.
- Unilateral nipple discharge.

c.   Bone.   2 marks
Brain.
Liver.
Lung.

d.   BRCA 1.   2 marks
BRCA 2.

e.   A mammogram would be appropriate for this lady as she will have 1 mark
less dense breast tissue than a young person.

13)

a.   Breast clinic.   1 mark

b.   Triple assessment.   1 mark

c.   Fine-needle aspiration.   2 marks
Core biopsy.

d.   Any 3 from: 3 marks
- Smoking.
- Alcohol.
- Poor nutrition.
- Obesity.
- Age >65 years.

e.   Any 3 from: 3 marks
- Diabetes.
- Vascular disease.
- Steroid use.
- Chemotherapy.
- Autoimmune disease.
- Hypoalbuminaemia.

- Infection.
- Ascites.
- Malignancy.
- Jaundice.
- Radiotherapy.
- Chemotherapy.

Chapter 14

Urology
ANSWERS

Single best answers

1) a.
2) c.
3) d.
4) b.
5) c.
6) a.
7) b.
8) c.
9) d.
10) a.
11) d.
12) b.
13) a.
14) d.
15) b.
16) a.
17) d.
18) c.
19) b.
20) c.

21) d.
22) a.
23) c.

Extended matching question answers

1) b

This description as "a bag of worms" on palpation is typical for a varicocele.

2) d

Torsion should always be considered for unilateral testicular pain. Key features include severe pain that is difficult to control and a high-riding testis with abnormal lie.

3) e

Epididymo-orchitis is inflammation of the epididymis and testes. It is often caused by infection such as a sexually transmitted infection or the mumps. Orchitis and parotitis may be associated with mumps.

4) a

These are typical examination findings with a hydrocele.

5) f

Testicular tumours may present with a painful or painless lump. A tumour is more likely in this case as the mass cannot be separated from the testis and has a gradual onset.

6) b

Painless haematuria should be investigated as suspected bladder cancer until proven otherwise.

7) f

This patient has acute urinary retention and this should be treated urgently with a catheter. As he has had haematuria beforehand, a possible cause would be clot retention so this would require irrigation.

8)   d

This patient has symptomatic anaemia as a result of his haematuria so he requires a blood transfusion.

9)   e

In this scenario, there is a clear cause for the retention (epidural) and haematuria (catheterisation) so no further investigation is required.

10)   h

This patient may have a recurrence of bladder cancer and requires the appropriate investigations for this.

11)   g

Penile cancers tend to be squamous cell carcinomas and a well-demarcated or ulcerated lesion should raise a suspicion.

12)   b

In paraphimosis, the retracted foreskin becomes swollen and painful, constricts the glans and may be difficult to replace.

13)   d

This patient has phimosis but the dry white appearance is typical of balanitis xerotica obliterans, a common pathological cause of phimosis.

14)   a

Phimosis is a tightness of the foreskin causing a difficulty or an inability with retraction of the foreskin.

15) c

The appearance described is typical for Peyronie's disease. This requires no treatment unless it is causing pain or disruption to function.

16) d

This patient has a urine dip suggestive of bacterial presence and her symptoms suggest infection.

17) a

This patient has mixed voiding and storage symptoms combined with a terminal dribble, suggestive of prostatic enlargement. This is likely to be benign although malignant disease should be considered.

18) g

This patient's previous history is suggestive of benign enlargement; however, haematuria and a raised PSA may indicate the presence of malignant disease.

19) b

An overactive bladder is caused by inappropriate detrusor contraction and this description is a common presenting complaint.

20) h

Poor stream in a young man is suggestive of a urethral stricture. Trauma to the perineum or pelvis is the commonest cause.

21) e

Proteus is associated with renal tract calculi, particularly staghorn calculi. CT is the gold standard for the detection of renal tract stones.

22) c

This patient has a simple UTI and is well and stable, and so could be treated with oral antibiotics.

23) g

This patient has recurrent culture-proven UTIs so this requires investigation as he is male. The first step should be a renal tract ultrasound followed by flexible cystoscopy.

24) h

In the absence of UTI symptoms and in a non-pregnant female, asymptomatic bacteriuria does not require treatment.

25) f

Sepsis and systemic features or symptoms of upper tract UTI require treatment with intravenous antibiotics.

26) d

Phimosis may be physiological at this age.

27) f

In hypospadias, the urethra may open anywhere in the midline from the glans to the perineum.

28) h

Torsion should be considered for an acute, unilateral onset of testicular pain, particularly in a teenage boy.

29) c

The testes would usually have descended by this age and persistent absence is more suggestive of cryptorchidism than retractile testes.

30) g

A transilluminable scrotum is suggestive of a hydrocele. A congenital hydrocele is caused by latency of the processes vaginalis so communicates with the peritoneal cavity, hence the swelling disappearing when supine as the fluid returns to the peritoneum.

31) c

This history is suggestive of torsion so this patient requires urgent surgery to investigate and treat a possible ischaemic testicle.

32) f

A hydrocele does not require any treatment routinely unless it is causing pain or affecting function. As the hydrocele is affecting exercise function, it should be surgically repaired.

33) a

Testicular tumours are biopsied by excision to prevent seeding of a malignant tumour. For this reason they are removed by an inguinal approach as the scrotal skin has different lymphatic drainage.

34) d

Gradual-onset pain and well-tolerated examination with a tender epididymis is more suggestive of epididymo-orchitis than torsion.

35) g

A new-onset left-sided varicocele should raise a suspicion of renal tumours as the left gonadal vein drains into the left renal vein, whereas the right gonadal vein drains directly into the IVC.

36) b

Painless haematuria should be treated as bladder cancer until proven otherwise. In tropical countries, SCC is far more common than TCC due to schistosomiasis.

37) e

Stasis of urine caused by incomplete bladder emptying may lead to the formation of bladder stones.

38) d

This history is typical for ureteric colic. In a 40-year-old, an AAA is possible but less likely.

39) a

Risk factors for TCC include smoking and exposure to certain industrial chemicals found in paints, dyes and rubbers.

40) h

Cystitis is not always infective and may be caused by radiation.

41) g

This history is very suggestive of ureteric colic and a CT KUB is the gold standard for stone detection.

42) d

This patient is septic and requires urgent decompression of his renal tract, usually by nephrostomy or stent insertion.

43) h

This stone is too large to pass down the ureter but as it is causing a problem, this requires treatment. A percutaneous nephrolithotomy will allow direct access to the stone in the renal pelvis and ideally should take place in the absence of infection.

44) a

Stones of under 5mm will usually pass on their own.

45) e

Due to its size, this stone is less likely to pass without intervention. This patient is stable but in pain so the stone may be treated primarily if there is no evidence of infection.

Short answer question answers

1)

a. Abdominal aortic aneurysm.   1 mark

b. Non-contrast CT of the renal tract (CT KUB).   1 mark

c. Any 3 from: 3 marks
- Calcium oxalate.
- Uric acid.
- Calcium phosphate.
- Struvite.
- Cystine.

d. Pelvic-ureteric junction.   3 marks
Vesico-ureteric junction.
Pelvic brim.

e. Any 1 of: 2 marks
- Conservative management: lifestyle advice, analgesia.
- Non-operative management: nephrostomy, lithotripsy.
- Operative management: stenting, ureteroscopic removal.

2)

a. Pyelonephritis.   1 mark

b. Urine dip.   3 marks
Blood tests.
MSU culture.

c. Any 2 from: 2 marks
- Frequency of urine.
- Urgency of urine.
- Dysuria.
- Abdominal pain.
- Fever.
- Chills.
- Rigors.
- Malaise.

d.   Any 3 from: 3 marks
  ● Female.
  ● Stone disease.
  ● Enlarged prostate.
  ● Urethral stricture.
  ● Indwelling catheter.
  ● Urinary retention.
  ● Elderly.
  ● Diabetes.
  ● Immunosuppression.

e.   Antibiotics: 3 days for an uncomplicated UTI; 7-10 days for a   1 mark
     complicated UTI.

3)
a.   Full history and examination.   3 marks
     Testicular ultrasound.
     Tumour markers: beta HCG, α-fetoprotein, LDH.
b.   Seminomas and non-seminomatous germ cell tumours.   1 mark
c.   Lymphatic spread to the para-aortic lymph nodes.   1 mark
d.   Ages 20-30: non-seminomatous germ cell tumours.   2 marks
     Ages 30-40: seminomas.
e.   Orchidectomy via the inguinal route is the mainstay of treatment.   3 marks
     Sperm banking should be offered before an orchidectomy.
     A CT of the abdomen and thorax for staging.

4)
a.   Storage: frequency, urgency, nocturia, dysuria.   2 marks
     Voiding: hesitancy, poor stream, dribbling.
b.   Benign prostatic enlargement.   1 mark
c.   Alpha-blockers, e.g. tamsulosin (1 mark), followed by 5-alpha-   2 marks
     reductase inhibitors, e.g. finasteride (1 mark).
d.   PSA is prostate-specific antigen. It is produced by the prostate as part   2 marks
     of its normal physiology (1 mark). Higher levels will be detectable

with larger prostates but increased levels disproportionate to the prostate size may be due to prostate cancer (1 mark).

e. Any 3 from: 3 marks
- Enlarged prostate.
- Bladder stones.
- Blood clots.
- Blocked catheter.
- Opioids.
- Spinal or epidural block.
- Anticholinergics.
- Tricyclic antidepressants.
- Alcohol.
- Neuromuscular disorders.

5)

a. Full history and examination.   3 marks
    Imaging of the renal tract.
    Direct visualisation of the bladder with flexible cystoscopy.

b. Transitional cell carcinoma is the commonest bladder cancer in the 1 mark
    UK.
    Squamous cell carcinoma is the commonest bladder cancer worldwide.

c. Any 2 from: 2 marks
- Smoking.
- Azo dyes.
- Beta naphthylamine.
- Schistosomiasis.

d. Conservative, e.g. symptom control or monitoring growth.   3 marks
    Surgical, e.g. surgical resection, diathermy, cystectomy.
    Adjunctive, e.g. radiotherapy, chemotherapy, immunotherapy.

e. TNM staging.   1 mark

6)

a. Catheterisation. 1 mark

b. His abdomen may be distended with a palpable bladder, dull to percussion. 1 mark

c. Bloods including U&Es to exclude electrolyte disorders and AKI. 3 marks
IV fluids.
Strict fluid balance monitoring.

d. Any 3 from: 3 marks
- Benign prostatic enlargement.
- Constipation.
- Morphine.
- Tricyclic antidepressants.
- UTI.
- Bladder stones.
- Prostatic adenocarcinoma.
- Neuromuscular disorders.

e. Transurethral resection of the prostate (TURP). 2 marks
Long-term catheterisation if surgery is not acceptable.

7)

a. Renal cell adenocarcinoma. 1 mark

b. Any 3 from: 3 marks
- Incidental finding.
- Loin mass.
- Visible haematuria.
- Sepsis.
- Pain.
- Metastases.

c. No. Biopsy risks seeding tumour into the peritoneum. 2 marks

d. TNM staging. 2 marks

e. Surgery is the main option with a radical or partial nephrectomy. For metastatic disease there are medical therapies available but these may be for palliative symptomatic relief only, e.g. radiotherapy for bone metastases. 2 marks

8)
a.   Testicular torsion.   1 mark
b.   Unilateral severe testicular pain.   3 marks
      High-riding testicle.
      Abnormal lie of the testicle, e.g. oblique or horizontal.
c.   Urgent exploration of the scrotum.   2 marks
      Orchidectomy if the testis is infarcted.
d.   Scrotal haematoma.   3 marks
      The risk of orchidectomy if the testicle is infarcted.
      The need for exploration and fixation of the contralateral side if a
      torsion is found.
e.   The testicular artery, a paired branch running off the abdominal aorta. 1 mark

9)
a.   Urethral stricture.   1 mark
b.   From proximal to distal: prostatic urethra, membranous urethra, 3 marks
      penile/spongy urethra.
c.   Any 2 from: 2 marks
      ●   Pelvic trauma.
      ●   Perineal trauma.
      ●   Sexually transmitted infections.
d.   Any 2 from: 2 marks
      ●   Haematuria.
      ●   Post-micturition dribbling.
      ●   Urinary retention.
      ●   Weak or divergent stream.
      ●   Difficult catheterisation.
e.   Dilatation.   2 marks
      Urethroplasty.

10)
a.   The presence of bacteria in the urine.   1 mark

b. The inflammatory response of the urothelium to bacterial invasion. 1 mark

c. No, as asymptomatic bacteriuria may be insignificant. 2 marks

d. Any 2 from: 2 marks
- *E. coli.*
- *Staphylococcus saprophyticus.*
- *Enterococcus faecalis.*
- *Proteus spp.*
- *Klebsiella.*

e. Any 4 from: 4 marks
- In children: loss of appetite, change in behaviour, failure to thrive, abdominal pain, new urinary incontinence in potty-trained child.
- In the elderly: delirium, decreased mobility, lethargy.

11)

a. Adenocarcinoma of the prostate. 1 mark

b. Prostate cancer tends to grow in the peripheral zone. 2 marks
Metastasis typically spreads to the bones and iliac lymph nodes.

c. TNM staging. Gleason score based on histology. 2 marks

d. PSA levels may be monitored on patients postoperatively to look for 3 marks recurrence of the cancer (1 mark), during or after adjuvant therapies to monitor suppression of the disease (1 mark) or for patients on active surveillance to indicate development of their cancer (1 mark).

e. Any 2 from: 2 marks
- Surveillance.
- Resection.
- Radiotherapy.
- Hormone therapy.

12)

a. Smoothly swollen hemiscrotum. 2 marks
Transillumination.

b. Hydroceles are conservatively managed if asymptomatic. If 2 marks symptomatic, they can be surgically repaired by reconfiguring the tunica vaginalis to prevent the accumulation of lymphatic fluid.

c.   Patent processes vaginalis.   1 mark

d.   A varicocele is a varicosity and engorgement of the veins of the   3 marks
pampiniform plexus (1 mark). There is fluctuant swelling that
increases on standing (1 mark) and it will not transilluminate (1 mark).

e.   This may be a presenting feature of a renal tumour (1 mark) as the left   2 marks
testicular vein drains into the left renal vein, whereas the right renal
vein drains directly into the inferior vena cava (1 mark).

13)

a.   Acute kidney injury.   1 mark

b.   Pre-renal.   1.5 marks
Renal.
Post-renal.

c.   Pre-renal: hypovolaemia, renal artery stenosis, sepsis.   1.5 marks
Renal: SLE, IgA nephropathy, Goodpasture's disease, acute tubular
necrosis, acute interstitial nephritis, acute glomerulonephritis,
vasculitis.
Post-renal: ureteric obstruction (e.g. by stone), urinary retention,
bladder outflow obstruction, ureteric injury.

d.   Pre-renal: volume replacement.   3 marks
Renal: control of underlying renal disease.
Post-renal: relief of obstruction by either a JJ stent, nephrostomy or
removal of the obstructing object.

e.   Any 3 from: 3 marks
- Refractory hyperkalaemia.
- Refractory pulmonary oedema.
- Severe metabolic acidosis.
- Uremic pericarditis.
- Uremic encephalopathy.
- Ethylene glycol intoxication.
- Methanol intoxication.
- Lithium overdose.
- Salicylate overdose.

Chapter 15

Neurosurgery
ANSWERS

Single best answers

1) d.
2) d.
3) b.
4) a.
5) c.
6) b.
7) d.
8) a.
9) c.
10) c.
11) d.
12) b.
13) a.
14) d.
15) b.
16) c.
17) a.
18) b.
19) d.
20) c.

21) b.
22) c.
23) a.

Extended matching question answers

1) a

   This patient is presenting with seizures and a focal left-sided neurology which has gradually progressed with no past medical history of note. This presentation is most consistent with a meningioma as these often present with seizures and focal symptoms affecting women more than men.

2) h

   The most common option for these symptoms of unilateral hearing loss and tinnitus is a vestibular schwannoma.

3) f

   This is most likely a pituitary tumour which is causing bitemporal hemianopia by its effects on the optic chiasm. The nipple discharge is galactorrhoea related to a hormone imbalance due to the tumour.

4) g

   This patient has known metastases and primary lung cancer. His presentation with neurological symptoms is most likely representative of cerebral metastases.

5) c

   The symptoms this patient is presenting with are of a raised ICP. Her presentation combines respiratory symptoms as well as neurology, and their background implies a risk of TB — making a tuberculoma the most likely option.

6) c

This presentation is classical for a subarachnoid haemorrhage — typically a 'thunderclap' headache of sudden onset which is described as the worst ever. It can also present with signs of meningism. The relevance of polycystic kidneys is the association of this condition with berry aneurysms — these are the most common cause of SAH.

7) h

Whilst the background of SAH would make you want to exclude this, the symptoms do not point to this as the most obvious cause in this case. These symptoms can be explained by hydrocephalus, which is supported by the CT scan findings of bilaterally dilated ventricles.

8) a

These symptoms are in keeping with a raised intracranial pressure. This can often be caused by a space-occupying lesion, bleeding, etc., but the normal CT scan makes these significantly less likely. The patient's age and background, along with a normal CT scan, support idiopathic intracranial hypertension (IIH).

9) e

This patient presents with unilateral symptoms which sound like they originate in the vestibular/8th nerve region. As such, a diagnosis of a vestibular schwannoma is supported.

10) b

This patient is presenting with symptoms and signs of a raised intracranial pressure and focal right-sided neurological symptoms. Given her age and lack of other available medical history, there should be a high suspicion of primary CNS malignancy. Of these, the most common is a glioma.

11) a

A history suggesting a raised ICP must prompt thoughts of space-occupying lesions or bleeds. This patient's background puts him at an increased risk of trauma. The history of fluctuating consciousness with nausea and vomiting are key features of a presentation of subdural haemorrhage.

12) d

This patient's symptoms sound initially like that of a stroke, particularly on a background of no trauma and no warning. Her symptoms have now completely resolved — as such this fits the criteria for a possible TIA.

13) f

This patient scores 10: E — opens eyes to voice (3); V — incomprehensible sounds (2); M — localises to pain (5).

14) c

This history of head trauma and unconsciousness followed by a lucid interval is fairly classical of an extradural haemorrhage.

15) h

This patient scores 12: E — opens eyes spontaneously (4); V — confused (4); M — withdraws to pain (4).

16) a

This presentation is of a thunderclap headache — often associated with an SAH. The CT findings support this.

17) d

This history is indicative of a raised ICP. The CT scan, however, does not appear to show any obvious pathology. This would indicate that a diagnosis of IIH is most likely.

18) c

The head injury and loss of consciousness should prompt a concern over serious intracranial pathology. The CT scan results showing a lens-shaped area of probable bleeding is indicative of an extradural haematoma.

19) b

The history indicates there may have been an intracranial injury. The persistent headache, along with CT evidence, may suggest some ongoing pathology. A crescent-shaped lesion on CT indicates a subdural haematoma, with a midline shift indicating significant pathology.

20) h

This presentation could initially be confusing as it involves multiple organ systems. These are, however, all features of hydrocephalus. The CT scan showing enlarged ventricles bilaterally supports this.

21) f

Pre-operative corticosteroids and anti-epileptic medications are often given prior to removal of meningiomas. These are surgically removed as they are chemotherapy-resistant. Radiotherapy may also be used.

22) a

Fluid resuscitation helps to maintain blood pressure and therefore cerebral perfusion pressure. The main aim of managing a primary brain injury or bleed is to avoid secondary brain injury due to hypoperfusion. Clipping or coiling is often done endovascularly to control and hopefully stop the bleeding.

23) c

A biconcave-shaped bleed implies an extradural haematoma. This is due to dural attachments to the skull which prevent blood travelling any further. Surgical evacuation is often required.

24) h

These are medical options for reducing intracranial pressure and can be used in cases of hydrocephalus.

25) h

If medical treatment fails, repeated lumbar punctures can be used to treat hydrocephalus by removing CSF. This poses risks of infection and bleeding however. Other treatment options include ventriculoperitoneal shunts and sometimes surgical resection of the inferior occipital bone.

26) a

This patient scores 7: E — opens eyes to pain (2); V — no response (1); M — withdraws to pain (4).

27) d

This patient scores 6: E — no response (1); V — incomprehensible sounds (2); M — abnormal flexion (3).

28) f

This patient scores 9: E — opens eyes to voice (3); V — incomprehensible sounds (2); M — withdraws to pain (4).

29) h

This patient scores 12: E — opens eyes spontaneously (4); V — inappropriate words (3); M — localises to pain (5).

30) b

This patient scores 3: E — no response (1); V — no response (1); M — no response (1).

31) d

This patient scores 15: E — opens eyes spontaneously (4); V — orientated (5); M — obeys commands (6).

32) f

This patient scores 12: E — opens to pain (2); V — confused (4); M — obeys commands (6).

33) h

This patient scores 6: E — opens to pain (2); V — incomprehensible sounds (2); M — abnormal extension (2).

34) a

This patient scores 3: E — no response (1); V — no response (1); M — no response (1).

35) b

This patient scores 14: E — opens spontaneously (4); V — confused (4); M — obeys commands (6).

36) a

The presentation of a thunderclap, sudden-onset headache associated with vomiting and meningism must prompt thoughts of an SAH, which is the most likely diagnosis in this case.

37) b

The combination of endocrine symptoms with signs of a raised ICP imply a hypothalamic-pituitary axis issue. As she is having symptoms of irregular or absent periods, as well as a difficulty in conceiving, a pituitary tumour is most likely.

38) c

Severe headaches can be difficult to diagnose. With an indication of papilloedema, implying a raised ICP, yet little on a CT scan, a diagnosis of IIH is most likely.

39) g

A history of seizure in a non-epileptic must raise the suspicion of a sinister pathology. The focal neurological symptoms also mentioned imply a focal CNS lesion such as a meningioma.

40) d

The bilateral symptoms are not common for a vestibular schwannoma; however, the brown spots indicate this may be associated with neurofibromatosis 2, which can cause bilateral vestibular schwannomas.

41) d

This history of infective sounding symptoms associated with headaches are concerning. The fact that the headaches have features of a raised ICP must lead to imaging of the brain and skull. Given the background it makes an infective source more likely and the lesion described on CT is typical of a cerebral abscess.

42) h

Given this patient has a background of trauma and is anticoagulated, an intracranial haemorrhage must be high on the list of differentials.

43) c

A headache showing signs of a raised ICP associated with known or previous malignancy is concerning. The CT findings also imply multiple discreet cerebral metastases.

44) a

Focal neurological symptoms as well as a headache with features of a raised ICP imply an underlying space-occupying lesion. Of the features and choices for this question, a meningioma is most likely.

45) f

Unilateral symptoms like this particularly affecting the hearing and facial pain must make one suspicious of CNS pathologies. In this case a vestibular schwannoma is the most likely cause.

Short answer question answers

1)

a. Enlarged third ventricle.   2 marks
   Enlarged lateral ventricles.

b. Any 2 from: 2 marks
   - Postural headaches.
   - Cognitive decline.
   - Confusion.
   - Gait disturbance.
   - Urinary incontinence.
   - Nausea.
   - Vomiting.
   - Drowsiness.

c. Cranial nerve 6 (abducens nerve).   2 marks

d. Any 2 from: 2 marks
   - Congenital malformation.
   - Post-haemorrhagic.
   - Post-meningitis.
   - Choroid plexus papilloma.

e. Any 1 from: 2 marks
   - Medical: furosemide, acetazolamide, repeated lumbar punctures.
   Any 1 from:
   - Surgical: resection of inferior occipital bone, ventriculoperitoneal shunt.

2)

a. 7. E — opens eyes to pain (2); V — incomprehensible sounds (2); M — abnormal flexion (3).   1 mark

b. Cushing's reflex.   2 marks

c.   Irregular respiration.   2 marks
     Death.
d.   Raised intracranial pressure.   2 marks
e.   Any 3 from: 3 marks
     ● Normothermia or mild hypothermia.
     ● Bed head raised to 30°.
     ● Treat seizures.
     ● Analgesia.
     ● Mannitol.
     ● Intubation.
     ● Decompressive craniotomy.
     ● Analgesia.
     ● Oxygen.
     ● Normocarbia.
     ● Sedation.

3)
a.   Battle's sign.   2 marks
b.   Any 2 from: 2 marks
     ● CSF rhinorrhoea.
     ● Racoon eyes.
     ● Hemotympanum.
     ● Reduced GCS.
     ● Cranial nerve palsy.
     ● Conductive deafness.
     ● Nystagmus.
     ● Vomiting.
c.   Protecting the airway as the GCS is less than 8.   1 mark
d.   Depressed skull fracture.   2 marks
e.   Halo test: dabbing the suspected material on tissue paper; if the halo   3 marks
     sign appears, it indicates the presence of CSF.

4)

a. Glioma. 2 marks

b. Right parietal lobe. 2 marks

c. Neurofibromatosis. 2 marks

Tuberous sclerosis.

d. MRI. 1 mark

e. Any 3 from: 3 marks

- Histological level of differentiation.
- How aggressive the tumour is.
- How likely it is to spread.
- How rapidly it will grow.

5)

a. Benign intracranial tumour of Schwann cells in the vestibular portion 2 marks
of the 8th cranial nerve.

b. Neurofibromatosis. 1 mark

c. Any 3 from: 3 marks

- Tinnitus.
- Vertigo.
- Nausea.
- Vomiting.
- Pressure sensation.
- Vestibular dysfunction.
- Cranial nerve deficit if large.

d. Conservative with annual imaging. 2 marks

e. Any 2 from: 2 marks

- Facial nerve injury.
- Vestibular nerve damage.
- Vascular injury.

6)

a. Ventricular dilatation.   1 mark

b. Any 3 of: 3 marks
- Papilloedema.
- Postural headaches.
- Cognitive decline.
- Gait disturbance.
- Urinary incontinence.
- False localising sign of 6th CN palsy.

c. Obstructive.   2 marks
Communicating.

d. Any 2 from: 2 marks
- Congenital malformation.
- Post-haemorrhagic.
- Post-meningitis.
- Choroid plexus papilloma.

e. Any 1 from: 2 marks
- Medical: furosemide, acetazolamide, repeated lumbar punctures.

Any 1 from:
- Surgical: resection of inferior occipital bone, ventriculoperitoneal shunt.

7)

a. Berry aneurysm rupture.   2 marks

b. Hyperdense area in subarachnoid space.   3 marks
Blood between ventricles.
Enlarged ventricles.

c. Fluid resuscitation to prevent cerebral hypoperfusion.   2 marks
Nimodipine to prevent vasospasm.

d. Any 1 from: 1 mark
- Endovascular coiling.
- Clipping of aneurysm.
- Open surgery to control bleeding.

e. Any 2 from: 2 marks
    * Hyponatraemia.
    * SIADH.
    * Obstructive hydrocephalus.
    * Persistent neurological deficit.
    * Rebleeding.
    * Cerebral ischaemia due to vasospasm.

8)

a. Temporal bone.   1 mark
b. Middle meningeal artery.   2 marks
c. Post-traumatic loss of consciousness (1 mark) followed by lucid   3 marks
    intervals (1 mark) and a gradual reduction in GCS (1 mark).
d. Biconvex (lens-shaped) area of high density (1 mark) limited by suture 2 marks
    lines (1 mark).
e. Surgical evacuation of haematoma.   2 marks
    Cautery of the suspected bleeding vessel.

9)

a. Bridging veins (1 mark) from the cortex to draining venous sinuses (1 2 marks
    mark).
b. Compression of the parasympathetic supply (1 mark) which travels on   3 marks
    the outer surface (1 mark) of the 3rd cranial nerve (1 mark).
c. Hyperdense crescent-shaped lesion on the inner surface of the skull.   2 marks
    There may be a midline shift or ventricular obliteration.
d. The colour of blood turns from hyperdense to isodense (1 mark) and   2 marks
    then to hypodense (1 mark).
e. Any 1 from: 1 mark
    * C-spine precautions.
    * Surgical evacuation of haematoma.
    * Lower ICP if raised with mannitol.
    * Nursing in upright position.
    * Airway protection.

10)

a. Prolactin.   1 mark

b. Bitemporal hemianopia.   2 marks

c. Tumour compression of the optic chiasm.   2 marks

d. Any 3 from: 3 marks
    - Prolactin.
    - GH.
    - ACTH.
    - TSH.
    - FSH.
    - LH.

e. Any 2 from: 2 marks
    - Diabetes insipidus.
    - Panhypopituitarism.
    - Visual field defect.
    - Obstructive hydrocephalus.

11)

a. 13. E — opens eyes to voice (3); V — confused (4); M — obeys   1 mark
    commands (6).

b. Cushing's reflex.   2 marks

c. 7-15mmHg.   2 marks

d. Mean arterial pressure.   2 marks
    Intracranial pressure.

e. Any 3 from: 3 marks
    - Normothermia or mild hypothermia.
    - Bed head raised to 30°.
    - Treat seizures.
    - Analgesia.
    - Mannitol.
    - Intubation.
    - Decompressive craniotomy.
    - Analgesia.

- Oxygen.
- Normocarbia.
- Sedation.

12)

a. 5. E — no response (1); V — no response (1); M — abnormal flexion   1 mark
    (3).
b. Decorticate posturing.   2 marks
c. Any 2 from: 2 marks
    - Serum electrolytes.
    - Blood glucose.
    - Toxicology screen.
    - CT of the head.
    - EEG.
    - ECG.
    - Lumbar puncture.
    - CXR.
    - Routine bloods.
d. Intubation to maintain a patent airway.   2 marks
e. Any 3 of: 3 marks
    - Pressure sores.
    - Long-term ventilation.
    - Infection.
    - Barotrauma.
    - Muscle wasting.

13)

a. Battle's sign.   1 mark
b. Racoon eyes.   1 mark
c. Base of skull fracture.   2 marks
d. Temporal.   4 marks
    Parietal.
    Sphenoid.
    Pterion.

e. Any 2 from: 2 marks
    - CSF rhinorrhoea.
    - Reduced GCS.
    - Cranial nerve palsy.
    - Conductive deafness.
    - Nystagmus.
    - Vomiting.

Chapter 16

ENT surgery
ANSWERS

1) d.
2) d.
3) a.
4) d.
5) a.
6) b.
7) a.
8) b.
9) a.
10) a.
11) d.
12) b.
13) c.
14) a.
15) c.
16) d.
17) c.
18) d.
19) c.
20) c.

21) c.
22) d.
23) b.

Extended matching question answers

1) g

   Ramsay-Hunt syndrome is caused by *Herpes zoster* in the geniculate ganglion. This leads to a vesicular skin rash, otalgia and hearing loss. These are associated with a lower motor neurone facial nerve palsy.

2) c

   Small children may not tell you that a foreign body is in their ear. A live insect in the ear can cause pain by movement or scratching/stinging.

3) a

   This is a classical presentation of acute otitis media. The most common causative organisms are *Streptococcus pneumoniae, Haemophilus influenzae, Moraxella catarrhalis, Staphylococcus aureus*.

4) e

   Nasopharyngeal tumours are more common in Chinese people, which appears to be multifactorial. They can cause ear pain which may be referred or due to direct invasion.

5) d

   Mastoiditis is an important complication of acute otitis media. It can lead to further complications such as meningitis, so it is important to recognise, as IV antibiotics and/or surgical management are required.

6) d

   Giving amoxicillin to patients with EBV infection frequently causes a generalised maculopapular rash.

7)   f

This patient has no signs of tonsillar inflammation.

8)   g

A swelling adjacent to the tonsil and uvular deviation suggest a quinsy.

9)   b

A food bolus usually presents after a meal, often with large amounts of meat. It can cause throat pain if it is at the upper oesophageal sphincter or chest pain if lower down.

10)   a

Deep neck-space infections may progress rapidly and can cause airway obstruction. A more serious infection is more likely in an immunosuppressed patient.

11)   h

A lump in the neck that moves on swallowing is likely to be in the thyroid.

12)   e

The short history and examination findings make a reactive node most likely.

13)   b

Cystic hygromas are lymphatic malformations that form cystic lesions. They are most common in the posterior triangle of the neck.

14)   e

The associated infective symptoms suggest these are reactive nodes.

15) d

This patient's age and the history of night sweats (a B symptom) mean a lymphoma must be ruled out.

16) d

Aminoglycosides are ototoxic and should be avoided in pregnancy.

17) a

A patient with unilateral hearing loss should always be investigated for an acoustic neuroma unless another cause is apparent. This also frequently causes balance problems.

18) g

Otosclerosis is a genetic cause of conductive hearing loss. It most commonly presents in middle-aged women with a family history of hearing loss.

19) b

Cholesteatoma is a rare complication of recurrent otitis media. It is an overgrowth of skin cells in the middle ear and needs referral to ENT as it is locally invasive and can cause significant damage to surrounding structures. The "brown flake" in this presentation is an attic crust, a classical sign of cholesteatoma.

20) h

In a patient of this age who is otherwise well with bilateral hearing loss, the most likely cause is age-related, or presbycusis.

21) b

In a child with stridor, epiglottitis should be considered. This child is unable to swallow saliva due to inflammation. Epiglottitis is much less common now due to vaccination against *Haemophilus influenzae* type B, but should still be considered, especially in children who have missed vaccinations.

22) f

Swallowing problems in this age group should be investigated for a malignant cause. In this patient, pharyngeal carcinoma is more likely than oesophageal due to the referred ear pain. This may occur via the glossopharyngeal nerve which supplies sensation to the tympanic membrane and part of the ear canal, but other common nerve supplies may also lead to throat pain being referred to the ear.

23) d

Patients with autistic spectrum disorders are more likely to ingest foreign bodies.

24) c

This patient has no other abnormalities found, so globus hystericus is most likely.

25) d

This child is suffering from lead poisoning due to redecoration releasing paint dust in an old house. This has caused pica leading to her ingesting a foreign body but has also caused the seizure. Pica has several causes which also includes iron deficiency.

26) a

Tinnitus in one ear combined with vertigo means an acoustic neuroma needs to be excluded. The patient may also have hearing loss but may not have noticed it, as it is unilateral. Menière's disease is less likely as it has been ongoing longer than a typical attack.

27) e

In the absence of any other symptoms and with the spacing between attacks, migraine is the most likely diagnosis. Migraines causing vertigo may occur without headache.

28) b

Rotational nystagmus is a sign of benign paroxysmal positional vertigo. Symptoms are often triggered by turning in bed.

29) h

Vestibular neuritis causes vertigo and nausea/vomiting. It is the same pathology as labyrinthitis, but it is more common for the nerve and not the labyrinth to be inflamed.

30) g

A sudden onset of vertigo in a patient of this age, particularly with cardiovascular risk factors, should be treated as a possible stroke unless other features are present that makes another diagnosis clear.

31) e

This child has epiglottitis, so the treatment is IV antibiotics. Nebulised adrenaline can be used to help keep the airway open. IV steroids may be used in some cases but oral steroids are not quick-acting enough.

32) f

This patient probably has a postoperative bleed which is causing swelling. This is resulting in airway obstruction and causes the widening of the neck. The surgeon should be called urgently to open the wound and relieve the pressure.

33) a

This patient has anaphylaxis caused by penicillin and needs adrenaline.

34) c

This male has developed airway obstruction caused by his cancer. In an emergency situation, a cricothyroidotomy can be performed to open the airway. A tracheostomy would be less appropriate as it would require going to the operating theatre and is a slower procedure.

35) b

CPR is needed as there is no evidence of breathing. See the Resuscitation Council choking algorithm for more information.

36) f

Swimming is a common risk factor for otitis externa.

37) a

Water pressure during diving can cause perforation of the tympanic membrane.

38) g

Otitis media is very common in children.

39) b

With a history of recurrent ear infections and foul-smelling discharge, a cholesteatoma should be suspected.

40) d

Malignant otitis externa is a form of otitis externa that can have serious consequences including osteomyelitis and cranial nerve palsies. It may present with non-specific features and is more common in immunocompromised patients, especially diabetics. This man should be admitted for IV antibiotics.

41) h

Vocal nodules occur due to overuse of the voice so are more common in professions such as singers and teachers.

42) e

The symptoms suggest malignancy and examination shows signs of a unilateral recurrent laryngeal nerve palsy. A laryngeal tumour large enough to cause vocal cord paralysis would be visible on nasoendoscopy so this is most likely to be a lung cancer.

43) g

Recurrent laryngeal nerve damage is a possible complication of a total or partial thyroidectomy. It may recover to varying degrees depending on the level of damage to the nerve.

44) d

This patient is young and also has pain, so inflammation of the vocal cords is most likely.

45) f

Slurred speech rather than hoarseness, as well as the sudden onset, suggests a stroke.

Short answer question answers

1)

a. Any 2 from: 2 marks
- Old age.
- Trauma.
- Anticoagulation.
- Trauma.
- Dry mucous membranes.

b. Little's area.   1 mark

c. A to E assessment (1 mark) and stabilise as needed. This may include   4 marks
fluid resuscitation (1 mark) and analgesia (1 mark). Pinch the fleshy
part of the nose and bend forward. The pressure needs to be applied
for 20 minutes (1 mark).

d. Any 2 from: 2 marks
- Packing.
- Cauterisation.
- Foley catheter.

e. Any 1 from: 1 mark
- Septal haematoma.
- Sinusitis.
- Deformity.
- Vasovagal episode.
- Aspiration.

2)

a. Any 2 from: 2 marks
- Dull tympanic membrane.
- Abnormal colour of the tympanic membrane.
- Retracted tympanic membrane.

- Air bubbles or air/fluid level seen behind the tympanic membrane.
- Loss of light reflex.

b. Any 1 from: 1 mark
- A hearing test (audiometry).
- Tympanometry.

c. Any 1 from: 1 mark
- Down's syndrome.
- Cleft palate.

d. Any 3 from: 3 marks
- Non-surgical: active observation, hearing aids, nasal auto-inflation devices.
- Surgical: grommets.

e. Any 3 from: 3 marks
- Poor speech development.
- Delay in learning.
- Social problems.
- Behavioural problems.

3)

a. Any 3 from: 3 marks
- Male sex.
- Smoking.
- Alcohol.
- HPV.
- Increased age.
- Poor nutrition.
- Occupational exposure, e.g. formaldehyde, asbestos.

b. Chest X-ray.   1 mark

c. The tumour will be removed with a wide excision margin to ensure all malignant cells are removed. As it has spread to local nodes he will require neck dissection to remove the affected lymph nodes.   2 marks

d. Adjuvant therapy is given after the tumour has been removed surgically, with the aim of destroying any remaining tumour cells. *1 mark*

e. Any 3 from: *3 marks*
- Infection.
- Bleeding.
- Scarring.
- Dysphagia.
- Malnutrition.
- Loss of voice.
- Fistula.
- Loss of taste.

4)

a. Any 1 from: *1 mark*
- A hearing test.
- Oto-acoustic emissions.
- Tympanography.
- MRI if unilateral to exclude an acoustic neuroma.

b. Endolymphatic hydrops. *1 mark*

c. Low-salt diet. *2 marks*
   Diuretics.

d. Any 3 from: *3 marks*
- Vestibular sedatives.
- Anti-emetics.
- Corticosteroids.
- Betahistine.

e. Any 3 from: *3 marks*
- Corticosteroids.
- Hearing aids.
- A Meniett® device.
- Vestibular nerve section.
- Labyrinthectomy.

5)

a. Any 2 from: 2 marks
  - *Haemophilus influenzae.*
  - *Streptococcus pneumoniae.*
  - *Moraxella catarrhalis.*
  - *Streptococcus pyogenes.*

b. Any 2 from: 2 marks
  - Young age.
  - Nursery/school attendance.
  - Smoking.
  - Down's syndrome.
  - Cleft palate.
  - Male sex.
  - Bottle feeding.

c. No immediate antibiotics.   3 marks
   Analgesia.
   Delayed prescriptions for antibiotics.

d. Any 1 from: 1 mark
  - Meningitis.
  - Hearing loss.
  - Mastoiditis.
  - Tympanic membrane perforation.
  - Intracranial abscess.
  - Facial nerve palsy.

e. Any 2 from: 2 marks
  - Any sign of complications.
  - Children under 3 months old.
  - Children aged 3-9 months with a temperature >39°C.
  - People systemically unwell.

6)

a. Parotid.   3 marks
   Submandibular.
   Sublingual.

b. Any 1 from: 1 mark
- Fine-needle aspiration.
- CT.
- X-ray.
- Sialogram.

c. Any 2 from: 3 marks
- Medical: compresses, massage salivary gland, hydration.

Any 1 from:
- Surgical: stone removal, gland excision.

d. Any 2 from: 2 marks
- Sjögren's syndrome.
- Bacterial infection.
- Viral infection.
- Radiotherapy.
- TB.
- Sarcoidosis.

e. Any 1 from: 1 mark
- Recurrence.
- Infection.

7)

a. Any 2 from: 2 marks
- 'Thick' voice.
- Swelling adjacent to the tonsil.
- Trismus.
- Snoring.
- Bulging of the soft palate.
- Tonsillar arch pushed forward.
- Deviated uvula.
- Erythema of arch and palate.

b. Hydration.   4 marks
Antibiotics.

Analgesia.

Steroids.

c. Any 1 from: 1 mark
- Aspiration of the abscess.
- Incision and drainage.

d. Any 1 from: 1 mark
- *Streptococcus pyogenes.*
- Group A *Streptococcus.*

e. Any 2 from: 2 marks
- Airway obstruction.
- Death.
- Deep neck-space infection.
- Mediastinitis.

8)

a. Any 2 from: 2 marks
- Tethering to surrounding structures.
- Firm consistency.
- Local lymphadenopathy.
- Ulceration.
- Blood/pus from the parotid duct.
- Bulging of the pharyngeal wall or soft palate.

b. Any 2 from: 2 marks
- CT scan.
- Fine-needle aspiration.
- Excision biopsy.

c. Adenoid cystic carcinoma. 1 mark

d. Any 4 from: 4 marks
- Facial nerve palsy.
- Infection.
- Bleeding.
- Scarring.
- Soft tissue deficit depending on the extent of the tumour.
- Frey's syndrome.

e. Superficial parotidectomy to spare the facial nerve.   1 mark

9)

a. CT of the head.   1 mark

b. Septal haematoma.   2 marks
    Urgent incision and drainage.

c. The patient should be seen in the clinic in 5-7 days to allow the 3 marks
    swelling to subside.
    Manipulation under anaesthetic 7-14 days after the injury.
    It can be done under local or general anaesthetic.

d. CSF leak. This can usually be managed conservatively.   2 marks

e. The haematoma should be aspirated as soon as possible. If this is not 2 marks
    done, avascular necrosis of the cartilage will result.

10)

a. A cholesteatoma is an overgrowth of keratinised squamous   1 mark
    epithelium in the middle ear.

b. Most cholesteatomas are acquired. Retraction of the tympanic   2 marks
    membrane causes indrawing of the pars flaccida. This allows
    squamous epithelium to grow inwards into the middle ear (1 mark).
    This process can also start due to trauma or surgical intervention such
    as grommet insertion (1 mark).

c. Any 2 from: 2 marks
    ● Discharge in the ear canal.
    ● Attic crust.
    ● Retracted tympanic membrane.
    ● Perforated tympanic membrane.

d. Any 2 from: 2 marks
    ● Hearing test.
    ● CT scan.
    ● Ear swab.

e.   Any 3 from: 3 marks
   - Facial nerve palsy.
   - Meningitis.
   - Abscess.
   - Deafness.
   - Recurrence.
   - Mastoiditis.
   - Sigmoid sinus thrombosis.
   - Labyrinthine fistula.
   - Osteomyelitis.
   - Chondritis.

11)

a.   In the fetus the thyroid gland develops in the foramen caecum at the   3 marks
   base of the tongue (1 mark). It then migrates downwards as the neck
   grows, forming the thyroglossal duct between the base of the tongue
   and the thyroid (1 mark). This normally obliterates, but if part of the
   duct remains patent, a cyst results (1 mark).

b.   Any 2 from: 2 marks
   - Fluctuant on palpation.
   - Moves upwards on protruding the tongue.
   - Non-tender unless infected.
   - Mobile.

c.   Ultrasound.   1 mark

d.   Any 3 from: 3 marks
   - Thyroid nodule.
   - Goitre.
   - Dermoid/epidermoid cyst.
   - Haemangioma.
   - Lipoma.
   - Pharyngeal pouch.
   - Basal cell carcinoma.
   - Squamous cell carcinoma.

e. Surgical excision.   1 mark

12)
a. Any 2 from: 2 marks
    - Protrusion of the ear.
    - Erythema and swelling over the mastoid process.
    - Otorrhoea.
    - Bulging tympanic membrane.
    - Sagging of the posterosuperior ear canal wall.
b. Mastoiditis is a complication of acute otitis media in which infection   2 marks
    extends into the mastoid air cells (1 mark) and may cause osteitis or
    periostitis (1 mark).
c. Any 2 from: 2 marks
    - Audiometry to assess hearing.
    - Bloods to assess inflammatory markers.
    - Tympanocentesis to aspirate the middle ear fluid for culture.
    - CT if there is diagnostic uncertainty.
d. Any 3 from: 3 marks
    - Antibiotics.
    - Mastoidectomy.
    - Myringotomy.
    - Tympanostomy.
    - Steroid drops.
e. Any 1 from: 1 mark
    - Facial nerve palsy.
    - Hearing loss.
    - Cosmetic issues.
    - Sigmoid sinus rupture.
    - Damage to the labyrinth.

13)

a. Viral.   1 mark

b. Any 3 from: 3 marks

    ● Reassurance.

    ● Analgesia.

    ● Warm compresses.

    ● Hydration.

    ● Safety netting.

c. Orbital cellulitis.   1 mark

d. Any 3 from: 3 marks

    ● Cavernous sinus thrombosis.

    ● Meningitis.

    ● Chronic sinusitis.

    ● Periorbital cellulitis.

    ● Subdural abscess.

    ● Sub-periosteal abscess.

e. Any 2 from: 2 marks

    ● Emergency admission for IV antibiotics.

    ● CT scan.

    ● Surgery to drain collection if antibiotics fail.

Chapter 17

Trauma and orthopaedics
ANSWERS

Single best answers

1) d.
2) c.
3) d.
4) b.
5) c.
6) a.
7) b.
8) a.
9) c.
10) b.
11) d.
12) a.
13) c.
14) d.
15) a.
16) b.
17) c.
18) d.
19) b.
20) d.

21) d.
22) c.
23) b.

Extended matching question answers

1) c

This is a rare form of cancer affecting children in the second decade of life. It is often metastatic at presentation and affects the pelvis, rib cage and metaphyseal proximal long bones most commonly. X-rays show a characteristic onion skin appearance.

2) g

It is a self-limiting synovitis common in 3-10-year-olds when they have a concurrent viral illness. The exact cause is unknown. It can cause a small rise in inflammatory markers and an effusion on USS.

3) h

The Kocher's criteria are used to diagnose septic arthritis. This patient meets all of these criteria which are: an inability to weight bear, febrile, a raised WCC and a raised CRP. He should be admitted for cultures, joint USS and aspiration +/- washout in theatre.

4) b

Osteochondritis dissecans — a joint condition whereby cracks form in the articular cartilage and subchondral bone.

5) a

A disease characterised by inflammation of the patella ligament at the tibial tuberosity. It mainly affects boys from 10-14 years old who are very active. They can have a painful lump over the tibial tuberosity.

6) a

This is often caused by a twisting injury and results in an immediate haemarthrosis because a small blood vessel runs within the ligament itself. It results in instability with a positive anterior draw test.

7)   d

This may present very swollen which may prevent you from feeling the classic 'step' in the tendon. Tears may be complete or incomplete. The gold standard for diagnosis is MRI but many hospitals still use USS. Early operative intervention is better as the tendon can retract significantly. Rehabilitation involves full weight-bearing in a knee brace which gradually increases the amount of flexion allowed in fortnightly increments.

8)   h

The presence of lipohaemarthrosis on aspiration should raise the suspicion of a fracture. CT would be the gold standard for follow-up. You may see a lipohaemarthrosis on plain film, in which case, joint aspiration should not be performed, as theoretically you will have turned a closed fracture into an open one.

9)   f

These often require surgical fixation if transverse or multifragmented. They are commonly fixed with a tension band wire. If it is a sheer vertical fracture and the extensor mechanism is intact, it can be treated non-operatively.

10) c

The usual mechanism of injury is a twisting type injury. Common symptoms include 'locking' of the knee whereby the torn fragment gets caught in the articular surface. It is confirmed by MRI and is often accompanied by an ACL or MCL injury.

11) e

A retrocaecal appendix can irritate the psoas muscle causing pain on right hip flexion. It is important to remember patients do not always present to the right specialty first time round.

12) a

A pathological fracture is a fracture through abnormally structured bone. This is not always metastatic, with Paget's disease and osteogenesis imperfecta being good examples of non-cancerous pathological fractures.

13) c

Perthes' disease is a form of osteochondritis which causes an interruption in the blood supply to the femoral head and leads to avascular necrosis. Classically, the child has a limp and painful internal rotation and abduction of the hip. It is bilateral in approximately 10%.

14) h

Psoas abscesses often present with pain on hip flexion in the context of sepsis. Intravenous drug users are at higher risk and *Staphylococcus aureus* is a common pathogen (which is prone to dissemination).

15) g

The usual treatment would include an ultrasound scan and if an effusion is present, an aspiration under general anaesthetic. MRI is widely used and treatment would include an extended course of intravenous antibiotics and washout in the operating theatre.

16) a

Bruised or isolated broken ribs are treated the same. Treatment is analgesia sufficient to allow deep breathing and coughing.

17) f

Good analgesia counselling when giving a prescription is imperative and NSAIDs should be taken for a limited period with PPI cover in selected patients (e.g. smokers, older people).

18) g

High-risk patients include those with long bone or pelvic fractures with associated vascular injury. The classic triad of symptoms include hypoxaemia, neurological disturbance and a petechial rash.

19) e

This is a diagnosis of exclusion and should always be taken seriously. This patient is clearly anxious and great care should be taken when counselling the patient prior to attempting procedures under minimal sedation. Respiratory alkalosis is common in hyperventilating patients and resolves quickly when the respiratory rate returns to normal.

20) b

The risk of MI is higher in older, frail patients when undergoing a general anaesthetic.

21) g

This fracture requires arthroplasty as treatment and this patient should be offered a total hip replacement. She is fit enough to cope with a longer anaesthetic and more involved rehabilitation.

22) c

This patient should be counselled on the risks and benefits of keeping his native hip vs. arthroplasty. He should be offered cannulated screws to preserve the native femoral head, with the main risk being avascular necrosis later requiring some form of arthroplasty.

23) d

This is an example of a pathological fracture. The fracture might be treatable with a DHS but with a likely distal lesion, she would be at risk of further fractures. She should be offered a long intramedullary nail to stabilise the femur.

24) f

This patient would benefit from a DHS. A short intramedullary nail would better control rotational forces if the fracture was in more than three parts, since it is fixed inside the bone rather than on the outside.

25) b

The fracture requires some form of arthroplasty; the patient may require something different. Leaving her with a broken hip and no operation will make nursing care incredibly difficult and painful so unless she is on the brink of death acutely, she should be offered an operation.

26) d

The fracture is dorsally angulated; therefore, it needs a dorsal slab. As the fracture is distal, she is unlikely to need an above-elbow cast to control rotational deforming forces.

27) e

A Bennett's fracture is an intra-articular fracture of the thumb base and can be treated in a thumb spica if it reduces in cast, otherwise it may need K-wire fixation.

28) a

Anything above the ankle generally goes into an above-knee cast, particularly if it's spiral in nature as rotation cannot be controlled unless the joint above and below are immobilised.

29) g

A Richard's splint is an extension brace which will support the knee but not allow any movement. You could use a range of movement brace if it was locked in extension. The patient can fully weight-bear but won't be able to lift their foot off the bed.

30)   f

Bilateral wrist fractures are a debilitating injury. Fixing her dominant wrist means you can treat her in a splint for 2-4 weeks. Bilateral POPs are heavy and the patient is likely to be very dependent on carers. There is a much lower threshold for treating a wrist fracture surgically if it is a bilateral injury for this exact reason.

31)   e

This is an example of a fragility fracture and is more common in this age group than an acute soft tissue injury because the bone is weaker than the soft structures. They classically bruise the whole arm and it is worth warning the patient. An effusion is visible and there is a painful but full range of movement, suggesting it is in the joint.

32)   b

This is suggested by his weakness in internal and external rotation. Given his age, previous occupation and length of history, this is likely to be a degenerative rather than acute cuff tear.

33)   h

This is common in people that work above head height such as hairdressers. Calcium deposits form most commonly in the supraspinatus tendon.

34)   d

This is often overdiagnosed but is common in people who overuse shoulder circumduction, such as bowlers and basketball players. It can be diagnosed with MRI and a labral repair can be performed arthroscopically.

35)   f

Ninety-five percent of shoulder dislocations are anterior. Posterior dislocations occur in epileptics or people who have been electrocuted. Given the short history, squaring of the shoulder and the fullness in the joint line, anterior dislocation is most likely rather than a frozen shoulder.

36) a

This presents with pain over the common extensor origin on the lateral epicondyle. It can be treated non-surgically with activity modification, splinting or platelet-rich plasma injection.

37) f

This is suggested by the acute mechanism and bruising. Weakness of supination is common and often forgotten about as biceps are the main supinator. It is often treated surgically if it is a full tear by sewing the tendon back onto bone.

38) e

The patient gives a history of a previous fracture and now being unable to straighten his arm. This can be managed surgically or non-surgically, depending on how much it interferes with his activities of daily living.

39) g

This is a palsy of the anterior interosseous nerve (a branch of the median nerve) which supplies flexor pollicis longus and flexor digitorum profundus to the lateral two fingers.

40) c

This is common in people who lean on their elbow, such as revising students. If infected it can be confused with an abscess.

41) b

This is usually caused by traction on an abducted arm with rupture of the lowest two nerve roots before or after they form the lower trunk.

It causes characteristic clawing of the hand due to palsy of the ulnar nerve and numbness in the C8 and T1 nerve distribution.

42) h

The posterior cord gives rise to both axillary and radial nerves. This will affect both shoulder abduction and wrist extension.

43) g

The median nerve travels down the middle of the forearm and may be directly or indirectly injured in penetrating trauma. Neuropraxia is the mildest form of nerve injury and symptoms may include paraesthesia and less than full strength in affected muscle groups. A stab wound in the antecubital fossa may cause weakness of wrist flexors and thenar muscles.

44) d

The radial nerve passes posteriorly around the humerus in the spiral groove before passing anteriorly over the lateral epicondyle. It can be injured in midshaft or spiral humerus fractures. This will cause weakness of wrist extension and finger extension.

45) a

This is caused by rupture of the upper trunk. It is characterised by internal rotation of the shoulder and extension and pronation of the forearm with a loss of sensation down the lateral aspect of the arm and forearm. It is commonly found in the neonatal period following a difficult delivery where the head and neck may have been forced away from the shoulder.

Short answer question answers

1)

a. Carpal tunnel syndrome is a condition whereby the median nerve is   3 marks
    compressed within the carpal tunnel (1 mark). Compression of the
    median nerve at the wrist leads to paraesthesia within the
    distribution of the nerve (thumb, index, middle and radial half of the
    ring finger) (1 mark) and weakness of the muscles supplied solely by
    the median nerve (abductor pollicis brevis) (1 mark).

b. Any 2 from: 2 marks
    - Women.
    - Diabetics.
    - Pregnant women.
    - Hypothyroidism.
    - Acromegaly.

c. Night splints to hold the wrist in a neutral position.   3 marks
    Steroid injections.
    Carpal tunnel decompression.

d. Any 2 from: 1 mark
    - Recurrence.
    - Complex regional pain syndrome.
    - Numbness over scar and thenar eminence.
    - Pillar pain (deep pain in the palm of the hand felt when carrying
      something heavy).

e. Nerve conduction studies will confirm if the median nerve has slowed   1 mark
    conduction and may explain her symptoms.

2)

a. Three joints: radiocapitular joint, proximal radioulnar joint and   4 marks
    ulnohumeral joint.

b.   Supracondylar fracture.   1 mark

c.   The median nerve. It runs down the middle of the forearm in both an   1 mark
anteroposterior and lateral view.

d.   Yes. There are a few concerning features in her presentation and   2 marks
although the history may not make you think of non-accidental injury,
there are suggestions of neglect. Namely, the delayed presentation
with a clear injury, presentation with someone other than a parent, a
suggestion that she had complained to her care givers but they were
not concerned. The paediatric team should be involved and the
named consultant for paediatric safeguarding.

e.   Any 2 from: 2 marks
- Cubitus varus deformity.
- Ulnar nerve palsy.
- Limited extension or pronation/supination.
- The carrying angle.
- Compartment syndrome.
- Volkmann's contractures.

3)

a.   Any 2 from: 2 marks
- Subchondral cysts.
- Osteosclerosis.
- Osteophytes.
- Joint space narrowing.

b.   Unicompartmental arthroplasty.   1 mark

c.   Any 2 from: 2 marks
- Loosening of the prosthesis within the cement.
- Damage to polymer liners.
- Infection.
- Periprosthetic fracture.

d.   Any 3 from: 3 marks
- IV access.
- Blood tests.

- Blood cultures.
- Knee X-ray.
- Knee aspirate in theatre.
- Antibiotics if unstable.

e. Any 2 from: 2 marks
- Analgesia.
- Physiotherapy.
- Revision arthroplasty.

4)

a. Any 1 from: 1 mark
- Nicotine constricts vascular smooth muscle impairing healing.
- Higher rate of non-union fracture.

b. Any 2 from: 2 marks
- Increased risk of infection.
- Poor wound healing.
- Increases risk of wound dehiscence.

c. Any 2 from: 2 marks
- Perform another X-ray to check ankle is still reduced.
- Application of an external fixation device if the position is not optimised.
- Definitive fixation after several days.

d. Any 3 from: 3 marks
- Focused history.
- Assess for neurovascular deficit.
- Remove cast.
- Measure compartment pressures.

e. Immediate fasciotomy.   2 marks

5)

a. Any 3 from: 2 marks
- Transient tenosynovitis.
- Septic arthritis.

- Malignancy.
- Slipped upper femoral epiphysis.
- Perthes' disease.
- Fracture.
- Osteochondritis dissecans.
- Osteomyelitis.
- Juvenile idiopathic arthritis.
- Avascular necrosis of the femoral head.

b. Typically affects boys between 4-8 years old.   1 mark

c. Flattening.   2 marks

Fragmentation of the femoral head as avascular necrosis occurs.

d. Any 3 from: 3 marks

- Blood tests.
- Urine dip.
- Blood cultures.
- X-ray.
- MRI.
- Lumbar puncture.
- Ultrasound.

e. Any 1 from: 2 marks

- *Staphylococcus aureus.*
- Group A *Streptococcus.*
- *Enterobacter.*
- *Haemophilus influenzae.*

Any 1 from:

- Long-term antibiotics.
- Bone biopsy.
- Draining subchondral collections.
- Debriding dead bone in the presence of persistent sepsis.

6)

a. Colles' fracture.   3 marks

Any 2 from:

- Extra-articular distal radius fracture.
- Dorsal displacement.
- Angulation.
- Radial tilt.

b. Any 2 from: 2 marks

- Sensory assessment of median, radial and ulnar nerves.
- Motor assessment of median, radial and ulnar nerves.
- Capillary refill time.
- Radial pulse.

c. Appropriate analgesia or sedation (1 mark). Counter-traction to   3 marks
exaggerate the deformity (1 mark). Steady traction to restore the
length before putting the wrist into slight flexion and ulnar deviation
(1 mark). Apply a dorsal backslab (1 mark).

d. Any 2 from: 1 mark

- Damage to neurovascular structures.
- Stiffness.
- Persistent pain.
- Prolonged recovery.
- Complex regional pain syndrome.

e. Any 1 from: 1 mark

- Patient living alone.
- Patient requiring help at home following injury.
- Dominant hand injury.
- Carer for another person.
- Medical cause for fall or injury.
- Other injuries.
- Open fracture.
- Neurovascular compromise.
- Joint dislocation.
- Compartment syndrome.
- Unstable fracture.

7)
a. Heberden's nodes.   2 marks
    Bouchard's nodes.
b. Any 2 from: 2 marks
    ● Ulnar deviation of fingers.
    ● Radial deviation of the wrist.
    ● Boutonnière deformity.
    ● Swan-neck deformity.
    ● Z-thumb deformity.
c. Any 2 from: 4 marks
    ● Non-surgical: analgesia, NSAIDs, steroids, splint, activity
      modification, biological agents, DMARDs.
    Any 2 from:
    ● Surgical: osteotomies, arthrodesis, arthroplasty.
d. An inability to actively extend the distal interphalangeal joint due to 1 mark
    an extensor tendon injury.
e. Thickening of the palmar fascia which eventually causes a fixed   1 mark
    flexion deformity.

8)
a. Tuberculosis of the vertebral body.   1 mark
b. Any 2 from: 2 marks
    ● Lytic destruction of the anterior vertebral body.
    ● Increased anterior wedging.
    ● Vertebral body collapse.
    ● Reactive sclerosis on a progressive lytic process.
c. The main route of transmission is haematogenous (1 mark). If two   3 marks
    adjacent vertebral bodies are affected, it usually spreads to the disc (1
    mark). The disc is avascular leading to caseous necrosis, loss of joint
    space and collapse (1 mark).
d. Avascular necrosis of the femoral head.   2 marks
    Osteomyelitis due to encapsulated organisms such as *Salmonella*.

e. Any 2 from: 2 marks
    - Congenital syphilis can cause several skeletal abnormalities including tibial bowing, saddle-nose deformities and teeth changes.
    - Disseminated gonorrhoea can cause septic arthritis.
    - Chlamydia can cause Reiter's syndrome.

9)

a. Any 2 from: 2 marks
    - Depth of glenoid fossa.
    - Glenoid labrum.
    - Rotator cuff.
    - Joint capsule.

b. Anterior dislocation.   2 marks
    Confirmed with a shoulder X-ray showing at least 2 views.

c. Any 3 from: 3 marks
    - Assess neurovascular status.
    - Physiotherapy.
    - Imaging to assess for a rotator cuff injury.
    - Support with a sling.
    - Sick note for work.

d. 71%. Accepted rule is 100-age = lifetime risk of redislocation.   1 mark

e. Any 1 from: 2 marks
    - Feeling of instability particularly in external rotation.
    - Pain.
    - Reduced muscle strength.
    - Stiffness.
    - Deformity of joint area.

    Any 1 from:
    - Hill-Sachs lesion resulting from forceful impaction of the humeral head against the anteroinferior glenoid rim.
    - Reverse Hill-Sachs lesion seen in posterior dislocation.

10)

a. The hip joint is formed by the femoral head and acetabulum (1 mark). **2 marks** It has a greater and lesser trochanter (1 mark). Posteriorly, these are joined by a crest (1 mark). The capsule attaches around the acetabular rim proximally and the intertrochanteric line and crest distally (1 mark).

b. The external iliac artery becomes the femoral artery as it passes **3 marks** beneath the inguinal ligament; this branches into the profunda femoris artery and superficial femoral artery. The profunda femoris artery branches into the medial and lateral circumflex arteries which anastomose around the femoral neck supplying the head in a retrograde fashion. A displaced neck fracture may damage and disrupt the blood supply of the surrounding vessels reducing blood supply which may lead to avascular necrosis.

c. Any 1 from: **2 marks**
   - ORIF with cannulated screws.
   - Arthroplasty.

   Any 1 from:
   - Fitness for surgery.
   - Able to participate in postoperative physiotherapy.
   - Pre-existing arthritis.

d. Total hip replacement, as the patient is a good surgical candidate and **2 marks** has an ability to participate in her own rehabilitation.

e. Cannulated screws require less than full weight-bearing initially. All **1 mark** other options are full weight-bearing following the operation.

11)

a. Any 2 from: **2 marks**
   - Immediate reduction to reperfuse hand.
   - Splint after reduction and recheck neurovascular status.
   - Defect should be covered with saline-soaked gauze and wrapped in a sterile bandage.

b. A Galeazzi type fracture is a distal radius fracture with a distal **1 mark** radioulnar joint dislocation.

c. Radial height should be 11mm (10-13mm acceptable). 3 marks
Radial inclination 22° (21-25° acceptable).
Volar tilt 11°.

d. The Galeazzi fracture is extra-articular and easily plated with a screw 2 marks
across the distal radioulnar joint (1 mark). The intra-articular
comminuted fracture is unlikely to achieve absolute stability in its
fixation and will rely on secondary bone healing. Stiffness and
traumatic arthritis are likely; this injury carries the worst prognosis (1
mark).

e. His left forearm (Galeazzi fracture) needs above-elbow 2 marks
immobilisation and a non-adherent dressing over the open defect.
The right forearm requires a dorsal backslab.

12)

a. Any 3 from: 3 marks
- Radial nerve.
- Median cubital vein.
- Biceps tendon.
- Brachial artery.
- Median nerve.
- Pronator teres.
- Brachioradialis.
- Posterior interosseous nerve.

b. Damage to the common flexor origin located on the medial 2 marks
epicondyle.

c. Paralysis of all intrinsic muscles of the hand, flexor carpi ulnaris and 2 marks
flexor digitorum profundus to the ring and little fingers (1 mark). The
higher the injury, the less the deformity in the hand, known as the
'ulnar paradox' (1 mark).

d. He may have injured the biceps tendon. 2 marks
It should be investigated initially with an ultrasound.

e. Any 1 from: 1 mark
    ● Lack of muscle strength.
    ● Stiffness.
    ● Chronic regional pain syndrome.

13)

a. Radiculopathy is pain due to compression of a single nerve root which   2 marks
    has exited from the spinal cord.
    Myelopathy is pain due to compression of the spinal cord.

b. Any 2 from: 1 mark
    ● Paraesthesia over the lateral leg, lateral malleolus, dorsum of the
      foot and hallux.
    ● Weakness of the muscles of the anterior compartment.
    ● Foot drop.
    ● Weakness of the hallux extension.

c. Ankle: S1/2.   4 marks
    Knee: L3/4.
    Biceps: C5/6.
    Triceps: C7/8.

d. L3: medial knee.   2 marks
    L4: medial malleolus.

e. Deep peroneal nerve.   1 mark

Chapter 18

Fluids and electrolytes
ANSWERS

1) b.
2) d.
3) c.
4) d.
5) a.
6) b.
7) b.
8) a.
9) c.
10) b.
11) c.
12) c.
13) a.
14) d.
15) c.
16) a.
17) b.
18) a.
19) d.
20) b.

21) c.
22) d.
23) c.

Extended matching question answers

1) c

   The obligatory volume of urine is approximately 500ml per day to remove various solutes from the body, but taking into account daily fluid intake, approximately 1500ml of urine is excreted every day.

2) a

   Most water entering the gastrointestinal system is reabsorbed. Loss may be increased in conditions such as vomiting or diarrhoea.

3) b

   An increase in insensible loss is seen in patients with a fever or there is an increased respiratory rate.

4) g

   The normal maintenance requirement of sodium is 0.9-1.2mmol/kg/day.

5) f

   The normal maintenance requirement of water is 25-35ml/kg/day.

6) d

   This solution contains less sodium than 0.9% sodium chloride and is the most physiological fluid.

7) e

   The concentration of both sodium and chloride is the same in 0.9% sodium chloride.

8) a

Hartmann's solution contains a small amount of potassium.

9) e

The concentration of both sodium and chloride is the same in a 0.9% sodium chloride.

10) g

5% dextrose contains 5g of dextrose per 100ml; therefore, in 1L there is 50g of dextrose.

11) b

Potassium has an intracellular concentration of approximately 140mmol.

12) a

Sodium is divided into approximately 50% in the extracellular fluid, 10% intracellular fluid and 40% in bone.

13) e

Although values vary slightly, potassium has an intracellular concentration of approximately 140mmol.

14) e

Although values vary slightly, sodium has an extracellular concentration of approximately 140mmol.

15) g

Intracellular calcium is tightly controlled given its importance in cell signalling. It is 1000 times more abundant in the extracellular fluid.

16) e

Hartmann's solution contains a small amount of potassium.

17) b

The previous use of 0.18% saline and 4% glucose led to several preventable paediatric deaths. A National Patient Safety Alert was issued to remove this solution from use to prevent fluid-induced hyponatraemia in children and the NICE guideline NG29 published in 2015 now advocates the use of isotonic crystalloids with 5-10% glucose.

18) h

Colloids are divided into albumin, dextrans, gelatins, hydroxyethyl starch and pentastarches. Gelatins such as Gelofusin® or Haemaccel® are prepared by hydrolysis of bovine collagen.

19) d

Normal saline is a hyperchloraemic solution; it reacts with water to produce HCl and NaOH which are a strong acid and strong base, respectively. As the normal level of chloride is 100mmol compared with sodium at 140mmol, the effect of adding normal saline which contains 154mmol/L of each electrolyte has a larger impact on the chloride level causing an increase in HCl leading to a metabolic acidosis.

20) g

If using type-specific blood, a cross-match must be performed before using blood. In emergency situations, O negative blood can be used.

21) e

Chvostek's sign is the tapping on the facial nerve in front of the tragus causing the facial muscles on the same side of the face to twitch due to tetany. Trousseau's sign is elicited by inflating a blood pressure cuff above the systolic blood pressure for at least 3 minutes; this will cause muscular contraction by flexion of the wrist, thumb and metacarpophalangeal joints with hyperextension of the fingers. This sign is more sensitive for hypocalcaemia than Chvostek's sign. These signs are both seen in hypocalcaemia.

22) e

A decrease in calcium causes a slower influx during the plateau phase of the cardiac action potential; therefore, prolonging this section and delaying the repolarisation of the heart. It is important to remember the differences in shape between nerve cells and cardiac myocytes to understand this concept.

23) b

Due to the increase in extracellular potassium, the electrical gradient between the intracellular and extracellular compartments is decreased which causes an increased action of myocardial potassium channels leading to faster repolarisation.

24) a

Many theories exist on the origin of U waves including repolarisation of the Purkinje fibres, but they are seen in hypokalaemia possibly due to the T waves becoming flattened or prolonged repolarisation of these fibres leading to U waves appearing more obvious.

25) a

Key findings in hypokalaemia are a prolonged PR interval, ST depression, small or inverted T waves and the presence of U waves.

26) c

Calcium raises the threshold potential for depolarisation which helps to counteract the rise in serum potassium.

27) d

The Society for Endocrinology advocates a standard treatment of 0.9% sodium chloride 4-6L over 24 hours and the use of bisphosphonates such as zoledronic acid 4mg over 15 minutes.

28) g

If a patient has symptomatic hyponatraemia, then hypertonic saline can be used but will require specialist input from the critical care team.

29) f

Sando-K® is a good alternative to the use of IV fluids with supplementary potassium.

30) d

The rise in sodium is most likely due to a fluid deficit and rehydration should correct this.

31) a

Loop diuretics act by inhibiting the $Na^+/K^+/Cl^-$ co-transporter in the thick ascending limb of the Loop of Henle; this can lead to hyponatraemia and hypokalaemia.

32) b

This class of drugs inhibit angiotensin-converting enzymes preventing the conversion of angiotensin II from angiotensin I. Common side effects include hypotension, hyperkalaemia, a persistent dry cough, dizziness and renal impairment.

33) b

Amiloride and spironolactone belong to a group of potassium-sparing diuretics. Amiloride works by inhibiting the epithelial sodium channel (ENaC) in the distal convoluted tubules promoting sodium loss whilst maintaining potassium levels. Spironolactone is an aldosterone antagonist acting primarily on the aldosterone-dependent Na^+/K^+ channels in the distal convoluted tubule.

34) a

Thiazide diuretics work by inhibiting the Na^+/Cl^+ channel in the distal convoluted tubule and inhibiting aldosterone activation of Na^+/K^+ ATPase at the collecting duct.

35) b

Digoxin acts by inhibiting the Na^+/K^+ ATPase pumps mainly in the myocardium. Digoxin toxicity can be reversed using the digoxin antidote formed from antibody fragments currently under the tradenames Digibind® or DigiFab®.

36) c

Failure of the kidneys to excrete potassium will lead to a rise in level causing hyperkalaemia.

37) f

Conn's syndrome results from excess production of aldosterone by the zona glomerulosa. Excessive secretion leads to hypernatraemia and hypokalaemia. Serum renin levels are low.

38) c

In renal failure, secondary hyperparathyroidism may be present as not enough vitamin D is converted to its active form to promote phosphate excretion, resulting in the formation of excessive calcium phosphate leading to a fall in serum calcium and a raised serum phosphate.

39) d

Milk-alkali syndrome is caused by over-ingestion of calcium and alkali substances such as antacids. This leads to a high serum calcium and can lead to renal failure.

40) a

Refeeding syndrome is associated with nutritional supplementation following a period of starvation or malnourishment. Prolonged malnutrition leads to protein catabolism and phosphate depletion. Introduction of carbohydrate leads to an anabolic state. Blood results may note hypophosphataemia, hypomagnesaemia, hypokalaemia, hyponatraemia, hypocalcaemia and hyperglycaemia.

41) f

Metabolic acidosis can be subdivided into those with a high anion gap or those with a normal/low anion gap. A high anion gap is due to acids which are not measured in routine testing such as lactate. Examples of a high anion gap include diabetic ketoacidosis, lactic acidosis, ingestion of salicylate, ethylene glycol and renal failure.

42) c

A metabolic alkalosis will show an increased pH, a normal or raised $PaCO_2$, a raised HCO_3^- and can occur in conditions such as vomiting.

43) e

A respiratory acidosis will show a decreased pH, a raised $PaCO_2$ and a raised HCO_3^-. The causative factor is usually an increase in ventilation. Renal compensation may occur in an attempt to return the pH to normal.

44) d

A respiratory alkalosis will show an increased pH, a decreased $PaCO_2$ and a decreased HCO_3^-. The causative factor is usually a decrease in ventilation. Renal compensation may occur in an attempt to return the pH to normal.

45) a

A low/normal anion gap metabolic acidosis is due to electrolyte disturbances. Examples include renal tubular acidosis and loss of bicarbonate ions through processes such as diarrhoea or vomiting.

Short answer question answers

1)

a. Any 1 from: 1 mark
- 0.9% sodium chloride.
- Hartmann's solution.

b. Blood transfusion. 1 mark

c. What fluid deficiency is present? 3 marks
Which fluid compartment needs to be replaced?
Latest electrolyte results from U&Es and what is the most appropriate fluid to give?

d. Any 3 from: 3 marks
- Urine.
- Faeces.
- Sweat.
- Respiratory tract.
- Skin.

e. 1 mark for each correct column shown in Table 18.1. 2 marks

Table 18.1

	0.9% sodium chloride	Hartmann's solution
Sodium (mmol/L)	154	131
Chloride (mmol/L)	154	111
Potassium (mmol/L)	0	5
Lactate (mmol/L)	0	29
Calcium (mmol/L)	0	2
Glucose (mmol/L)	0	0
Osmolarity (mOsmol/L)	308	278

2)

a. Any 3 from: 3 marks

- Dyspnoea.
- Raised JVP.
- Distended neck veins.
- Pleural effusions.
- Peripheral oedema.
- Crepitations.
- Hepatomegaly.
- Ascites.
- Tachycardia.
- 3rd heart sound.
- Right ventricular heave.
- Low-volume pulse.
- Poor peripheral perfusion.
- Hypotension.
- Displaced apex.

b. Any 1 from: 1 mark

- Chest X-ray.
- Echocardiogram.

c. Any 2 from: 2 marks

- Oxygen.
- Vasodilators such as GTN or isosorbide dinitrate.
- Diamorphine.
- IV dopamine in hypotensive patients.

d. Any 2 from: 2 marks

- Hyponatraemia.
- Hypokalaemia.
- Hypomagnesaemia.
- Dehydration.
- Hyperuricemia.
- Gout.

- Dizziness.
- Postural hypotension.
- Syncope.

e. TURP syndrome results from the use of hyposomolar irrigation fluid **2 marks** such as 1.5% glycine. The absorption of large volumes of this fluid by the prostatic venous sinuses leads to a rapid volume expansion which causes hypertension and reflex bradycardia (1 mark). The excessive absorption of fluid dilutes serum sodium leading to hyponatraemia, cerebral oedema and hypothermia (1 mark).

3)

a. Any 6 from: **3 marks**
- Chronic cardiac failure.
- Liver cirrhosis.
- Water overload.
- Nephrotic syndrome.
- SIADH.
- Reduced water intake.
- Excessive 5% IV dextrose.
- Diarrhoea.
- Fistula.
- Ileus.
- Obstruction.
- Fever.
- Excessive sweating.
- Burns.
- Addison's disease.
- Thiazide diuretics.
- Loop diuretics.
- SSRIs.

b. Any 2 from: **2 marks**
- Nausea.
- Anorexia.
- Headache.

- Malaise.
- Seizure.
- Confusion.
- Muscle weakness.
- Coma.

c. Any 4 from: 2 marks
- Urinary sodium.
- Urinary osmolality.
- Serum osmolality.
- U&Es.
- Echocardiogram.

d. Any 2 from: 2 marks
- Slow correct through fluid restriction.
- Demeclocycline.
- Treat the underlying cause of hypervolaemia.

e. Central pontine myelinolysis.   1 mark

4)

a. Hypernatraemia.   2 marks
    Hypokalaemia.

b. Cushing's disease is the ectopic production of cortisol produced by a   1 mark
    pituitary tumour. Cushing's syndrome is the effect of excess cortisol
    on the body regardless of cause.

c. Any 3 symptoms: 3 marks
- Dehydration.
- Thirst.
- Lethargy.
- Weakness.
- Confusion.
- Nausea.
- Anorexia.

Any 3 signs:
- Signs of dehydration.
- Confusion.

- Coma.
- Seizures.

d. Any 1 from: 1 mark
- Oral fluids.
- IV 5% dextrose.

e. Any 3 from: 3 marks
- Intracranial haemorrhage.
- Brain damage.
- Death.
- Cerebral oedema if corrected too rapidly.

5)

a. Hypokalaemia.   2 marks
   AKI.

b. Any 4 from: 2 marks
- Diuretics.
- Steroids.
- Pyloric stenosis.
- Intestinal fistula.
- Conn's syndrome.
- Cushing's syndrome.
- Insulin usage.
- Renal failure.
- Postoperative losses.

c. Any 2 symptoms from: 2 marks
- Muscle weakness.
- Cramps.
- Palpitations.

Any 2 signs from:
- Hypotonia.
- Hyporeflexia.
- Tetany.
- Arrhythmias.

d. Any 2 from: 2 marks
- AF.
- Long PR interval.
- Small/inverted T waves.
- U waves.
- ST depression.

e. Any 2 from: 2 marks
- Oral K^+ supplements.
- Hold diuretics.
- IV supplementation in fluids if nil by mouth.
- Correct magnesium if low.

6)

a. Hyperkalaemia and hyponatraemia.   2 marks
Addisonian crisis.

b. Any 4 from: 2 marks
- Blood transfusion.
- Renal failure.
- Hypoaldosteronism.
- Addison's disease.
- DKA.
- Metabolic acidosis.
- Burns.
- Rhabdomyolysis.
- Potassium-sparing diuretics.
- Beta-blockers.
- ACE inhibitors.
- NSAIDs.
- Potassium supplements.

c. Decreased P wave amplitude.   3 marks
Tall tented T waves.
Widening of QRS complex.

d. 10% calcium gluconate.   1 mark

e. Any 2 from: 2 marks
  - Nebulised salbutamol.
  - Insulin/dextrose.
  - Calcium resonium.
  - Haemodialysis.

7)

a. Hypercalcaemia.   2 marks
    Raised phosphate and raised alkaline phosphatase indicates the
    presence of bony metastasis.

b. Any 1 symptom for each category: 3 marks
  - Mild: polyuria, polydipsia, dyspepsia.
  - Moderate: constipation, anorexia, nausea.
  - Severe: abdominal pain, lethargy.

    Any 1 sign for each category:
  - Mild: mild cognitive impairment.
  - Moderate: muscle weakness.
  - Severe: dehydration, arrhythmias, coma.

c. Any 2 from: 2 marks
  - IV 0.9% sodium chloride.
  - IV bisphosphonates.
  - Haemodialysis.

d. Any 1 from: 1 mark
  - Parathyroid adenoma.
  - Multiple gland hyperplasia.
  - Parathyroid carcinoma.
  - Multiple endocrine neoplasia (MEN) Type 1 or 2A.

e. Raised PTH.   2 marks
    Raised calcium.

8)

a. Hypocalcaemia secondary to removal of the parathyroid glands. 2 marks

b. Any 3 from: 3 marks
- Chvostek's sign (tapping over the facial nerve producing a spasm).
- Trousseau's sign (inflation of BP cuff causes a carpopedal spasm).
- If hypocalcaemia is chronic, this can cause abnormal dentition.
- Subcapsular cataract.
- Papilloedema.
- Confusion.
- Ectopic calcification.

c. Magnesium.   1 mark

d. Prolonged QT.   2 marks
Prolonged ST interval.

e. Any 2 from: 2 marks
- Vitamin D deficiency.
- Pseudohypoparathyroidism.
- Hypomagnesaemia.
- Rickets.
- Fanconi's syndrome.

9)

a. Uncompensated metabolic alkalosis.   2 marks

b. Any 3 from: 3 marks
- Vomiting.
- Diarrhoea.
- Diuretics (decreased K^+).
- Burns.
- Ingestion of base, e.g. milk-alkali syndrome.
- NG aspiration.
- Hypokalaemia.
- Barter's syndrome.
- Gitelman syndrome.
- Liddle syndrome.
- Cushing's syndrome.

- Conn's syndrome.
- Aminoglycoside toxicity.

c. Any 2 from: 2 marks
- Hypoventilation.
- Chvostek's sign.
- Trousseau's sign.
- Confusion.
- Cyanosis.

d. Any 1 from: 1 mark
- Hypocalcaemia.
- Organ failure.
- Shock.
- Coma.
- Atrioventricular tachycardias.

e. Respiratory compensation by decreased ventilation to retain carbon   2 marks
dioxide.
Renal compensation by increased excretion of bicarbonate.

10)

a. Uncompensated metabolic acidosis.   2 marks

b. Any 2 from: 1 mark
- Diarrhoea.
- Addison's disease.
- Renal tubular acidosis.
- Pancreatic fistula.
- Sepsis.
- Salicylates.
- Lactic acid.
- Ketones.
- Starvation.
- Renal failure.
- Ethylene glycol ingestion.
- Acetazolamide.

c. Any 2 symptoms from: *3 marks*
  - Fatigue.
  - Headache.
  - Confusion.
  - Lack of appetite.

  Any 1 sign from:
  - Tachycardia.
  - Jaundice.
  - Rapid and shallow breathing.

d. $Na^+ + K^+ - (Cl^- + HCO_3^-)$.   *1 mark*

e. Any 3 from: *3 marks*
  - Normal anion gap: diarrhoea, Addison's disease, renal tubular acidosis, pancreatic fistula, drugs such as acetazolamide.

  Any 3 from:
  - Raised anion gap: lactic acid, ketones, renal failure, ethylene glycol ingestion, salicylates, sepsis, starvation.

11)

a. Uncompensated respiratory acidosis with hypoxia and hypercapnia.   *3 marks*

b. Any 2 causes from: *2 marks*
  - COPD.
  - Severe asthma.
  - Drug overdose: opiates, benzodiazepines.
  - CVA.
  - Duchenne muscular dystrophy.
  - Myasthenia gravis.
  - Flail chest.
  - Kyphoscoliosis.
  - Pickwickian syndrome.

c. Any 1 from: *1 mark*
  - Anxiety.
  - Dyspnoea.

d.   Any 2 from: 2 marks
   - Shock.
   - Cardiac arrest.
   - Death.

e.   Type 1: normal or low $PaCO_2$ with a low PaO_2 (<8kPa/60mmHg).   2 marks
   Type 2: raised $PaCO_2$ (>6.5kPa/50mmHg) and a low PaO_2.

12)

a.   Compensated respiratory alkalosis.   2 marks
b.   Any 3 from: 3 marks
   - Anxiety.
   - Hysteria.
   - Pain.
   - Stimulation of respiratory centre.
   - Altitude.
   - Pneumonia.
   - PE.
   - Fever.
   - Head injury.
   - Stroke.
   - Pneumonia.
   - Pulmonary oedema.

c.   Any 1 symptom: 2 marks
   - Light-headedness.
   - Paraesthesia.
   Any 1 sign:
   - Visual disturbance.
   - Anxiety.
   - Restless patient.

d.   Any 1 from: 1 mark
   - Cardiac arrest.
   - Arrhythmias.
   - Tetany.
   - Seizures.

e. Any 2 from: 2 marks
    ● Reduced renal excretion of hydrogen ions.
    ● Increased urinary bicarbonate excretion.
    ● In the acute phase, intracellular buffering is responsible for a
      slight compensation.

13)
a. Any 4 from: 4 marks
    ● Idiopathic.
    ● Endocrine: hypothyroidism, Addison's disease.
    ● Ectopic production: small cell lung cancer, lung abscess, TB.
    ● Malignancy: lung, pancreas, ovary, lymphoma, thymoma.
    ● CNS: tumour, trauma, infection, stroke, multiple sclerosis,
      Guillain-Barré syndrome, meningitis, encephalitis, subarachnoid
      haemorrhage.
    ● Drugs: SSRIs, TCAs, opiates, haloperidol, MAOIs, diuretics,
      NSAIDs.
b. Inappropriate antidiuretic hormone secretion leading to water   2 marks
    retention and relative hyponatraemia.
c. A raised urinary sodium >20mmol/L and a raised urinary osmolality. 2 marks
d. Demeclocycline is usually used which is an ADH antagonist.   1 mark
e. Central pontine myelinolysis.   1 mark